D0160475

The Hormone Secret

The Hormone Secret

DISCOVER EFFORTLESS WEIGHT LOSS AND
RENEWED ENERGY IN JUST 30 DAYS

Tami Meraglia, MD

Foreword by Daniel G. Amen, MD

ATRIA BOOKS

NEW YORK • LONDON • TORONTO • SYDNEY • NEW DELHI

This publication contains the opinions and ideas of its author. It is intended to provide help-ful and informative material on the subjects addressed in the publication. It is sold with the understanding that the author and publisher are not engaged in rendering medical, health, or any other kind of personal professional services in the book. The reader should consult his or her medical, health, or other competent professional before adopting any of the sug-gestions in this book or drawing inferences from it.

ATRIA BOOKS

An Imprint of Simon & Schuster, Inc.
1230 Avenue of the Americas
New York, NY 10020

Copyright © 2015 by Tami Meraglia

All rights reserved, including the right to reproduce this book or portions thereof in any form whatsoever. For information, address Atria Books Subsidiary Rights Department, 1230 Avenue of the Americas, New York, NY 10020.

First Atria Books hardcover edition April 2015

ATRIA BOOKS and colophon are trademarks of Simon & Schuster, Inc.

For information about special discounts for bulk purchases, please contact Simon & Schuster Special Sales at 1-866-506-1949 or business@simonandschuster.com.

The Simon & Schuster Speakers Bureau can bring authors to your live event. For more information or to book an event, contact the Simon & Schuster Speakers Bureau at 1-866-248-3049 or visit our website at www.simonspeakers.com.

Designed by Paul Dippolito

Manufactured in the United States of America

10 9 8 7 6 5 4 3 2 1

Library of Congress Cataloging-in-Publication Data
Meraglia, Tami.
    The hormone secret : discover effortless weight loss and renewed energy in just 30 days / by Tami Meraglia, MD.
        pages cm
    "Atria nonfiction original hardcover."
    Includes bibliographical references and index.
    1. Women—Health and hygiene. 2. Weight loss. 3. Hormones. I. Title.
    RA778.M4858 2015
    613.2082—dc23
                            2014041501

ISBN 978-1-4767-6650-8
ISBN 978-1-4767-6652-2 (ebook)

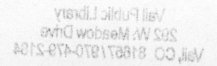

To the three most important women in my life: my mum, Elaine Casey, and my two daughters, Morgan and Kasey. There are no words to express the depth of my love.

Contents

Foreword

Tami Meraglia, MD, is a physician with a passion: to help women take charge of their own hormone health and happiness. Her unique voice is sorely needed today, more than ever, as women face hormone imbalances and deficiencies before, during, and after menopause. These conditions, which can diminish quality of life, are nothing new. What *is* new is that they are appearing earlier and when women are already stretched to the limit.

The scary truth is that women are often misdiagnosed by the medical establishment. Much is still misunderstood about the role of hormones in the female body, and how hormones affect the brain, bones, mood, weight, and general health. Dismissed by their regular doctors as simply tired or overworked, many of Dr. Meraglia's patients turn to her looking for answers. Their lives are often transformed by her holistic approach. Rather than viewing diseases as separate entities and automatically treating them with drugs, she focuses on the patient as a whole, believing in natural solutions as a first resort. She examines not only test results, but how patients look, feel, and function in our 24/7 society. Her mission is to help women be their best with simple changes in nutrition, attitude, and lifestyle.

Equally important is her ability to connect with patients as a woman, a wife and mother, and a daughter caring for elderly parents. I first met Dr. Meraglia after one of my PBS Specials. She reached out to me because she wanted to help her patients—and women on a larger scale—by writing a book to get the word out about the little-known effect of testosterone on female health. She wants to help women regain their energy, vitality, focus, and performance edge as they age.

I've seen her skills in action when we share the stage at speaking engagements. Dr. Meraglia electrifies the room with her down-to-earth advice, knowledge, and sense of humor. She understands women who are multitasking their way through life because she is one of them. She knows the stresses and strains women experience today because she has faced them herself.

There is no lack of information available on women's hormones. What is lacking is an effective system to achieve hormone balance and health in our society. In *The Hormone Secret,* Dr. Meraglia provides such a plan. This is a book about convenience for busy women in a world of change. Dr. Meraglia offers options, knowledge, and tools women have never had before. You couldn't be in better hands.

Daniel G. Amen, MD
Founder, Amen Clinics

Introduction

Have you gained weight in recent years even though your eating habits and activity level haven't changed? Has your waist expanded along with your jeans size? Do you wake in the morning more tired than you were when you went to bed? Do you crash at 3 p.m. every day, barely keeping your drooping eyes open? Are your arms flabby despite regular workouts with weights and machines at the gym? Do you notice memory problems and loss of focus, a feeling that you're losing your edge? Do you have osteoporosis or osteopenia?

Patients over forty tell me almost daily that they've gone to the doctor because they have such symptoms. They're tired and cranky; they don't sleep well or care much about sex. They're not as sharp as they used to be. They've added pounds and lost muscle. They make an appointment for a physical exam and a series of blood tests, and the results fall in the range of "normal." The doctor says, "You're fine," and suggests an antidepressant or sleeping pills or both.

Yet these women don't feel "fine." I am an MD board-certified in natural medicine, and an expert in hormone and aesthetic medicine. When patients come to my clinic in Seattle, Washington, for help, I tell them "normal" is a setting on a dryer, not an accurate description of your state of health. These patients simply don't have a condition or disease that is associated with a code that can be billed to insurance. Sometimes they're even diagnosed as the "worried well." Yes, there is a code for that! But the absence of disease does not equal wellness. Optimal health includes energy and vitality, and true prevention of conditions associated with aging.

You don't need to accept the slow decline of energy, mental clarity, and zest for life as the years go by. You don't have to accept waking up at 2 a.m. unable to go back to sleep. It isn't "normal." I don't want you to feel "fine." I want you to feel fabulous. And I'm going to show you how.

How Did We Get Here?

Chalk it up to the great hormone decline. The fact is, women's quality of life has changed dramatically in recent decades. Yes, we've been freed to achieve and realize our dreams as never before. But the educational and career opportunities, and the choices we now have in how and when we build our families, all come at a price. We're drowning in our increased responsibilities and the pressures of our multiple roles. We've also been slammed by a major blow to our hormone levels. It's a fact of life that hormone levels naturally decline as part of menopause and the aging process. Our mothers and grandmothers experienced these changes as well. But over the last thirty years these levels have dropped much earlier in women's lives and to a greater degree than ever before. Research shows that hormone levels now decrease 30 percent to 50 percent between the ages of twenty and forty alone. The result is an onslaught of hormone imbalances and deficiencies that weaken our ability to look, feel, and function at our best.

This hormone loss has accelerated, in part, due to the explosion of stress in our lives and to enormous environmental changes. Since the end of World War II, more than twenty thousand chemicals and other agents have been introduced into the environment and into our food system. You've heard about and read about it, yet chances are you haven't realized the extent of these changes. Most of the cleaning supplies under your sink contain chemicals that negatively affect your hormone levels. Hormones are put into poultry and cattle to fatten them up before they go to market, and that directly affects you. Pesticide residue on fruits and vegetables has an impact on your hormone levels. Chemicals used in canned goods and plastic containers throw off your hormones. All of these are called "hormone disrupters," or xenobiotics. Over time, they cause your hormone levels to drop faster than they ordinarily would.

But the No. 1 culprit above all the rest is stress. Stress is like a little Pac-Man, running through your bloodstream "eating" all your hormones. Stress, and the inflammation it creates, depletes your hormones and encourages development of diseases including cancer. Our 24/7 lifestyle and the ever-changing world we live in has taken a huge toll. We have heavier workloads, and even our play is not restorative. Our cell phones and iPhones and the demands they make accompany us on vacations at the beach, to the dinner table at meals, and sometimes even in bed. How many of us check our emails before getting out of bed in the morning? I know I am guilty. We have no true "breaks." No wonder our bodies are exhausted.

I've written this book to tell you about a true secret weapon that changes everything. It's one particular hormone that's the missing link to a better body, brain, and life. You won't believe the difference it can make. That hormone is testosterone. I'm not talking about taking this hormone. I'm talking about using nutrition, lifestyle changes, and supplements available over the counter to lose weight, look and feel great, and perform at your best. By following my 30-Day Plan, you actually can have enough testosterone in your body without medication—and the results are dramatic.

What Are Hormones, Anyway?

If you're like most women, you probably know very little about hormones, which can make or break the quality of your life after forty.

It's my job to educate you and demystify hormones, which are chemical messengers that control or regulate metabolism and many other body functions, and affect almost all organs. Deficiencies and imbalances in hormones make an impact on everything from your brain and cardiovascular system to your energy level, sleep cycle, skin, weight, sex life, and even your hair and nails. Hormones perform a lot like a symphony, where one instrument off-key can ruin the entire performance. If the level of one hormone is too low or too high, it affects the functioning of other hormones. For optimal health, your hormones must be restored to balance.

The key hormones for women include "the big three": estrogen, progesterone, and testosterone, and certain others. Estrogen and progesterone are known as "the sex hormones" for women, and levels of both drop dramatically in perimenopause and menopause. Estrogen deficiency causes hot flashes and night sweats, dries up your sex life (literally), and affects memory and mood. Low estrogen levels also cause irritability and can wreck your sense of well-being.

Progesterone is "the peaceful hormone." It calms you, reduces anxiety, and helps you sleep. Low levels of progesterone drain your energy and can cause anger-control problems and frustration.

Testosterone, my special focus in this book, is known as "the male hormone." But you have a small quantity of testosterone in your body, too (although men's levels are twenty times higher). That minimal amount you do have packs a powerful punch, playing an outsized role in your quality of life. Depletion of your testosterone levels as you get older is a life changer you can't afford. Yet testosterone and its benefits for women have virtually been ignored in traditional medicine.

The Testosterone Powerhouse

Testosterone helps you lose weight and firm up your body by building muscle and changing your muscle-fat ratio. Testosterone also helps build your bones. It's no accident that men are at much lower risk for osteoporosis than we are. Their higher testosterone levels give them an advantage. Testosterone also nourishes your brain, which may be a reason men are at much lower risk for Alzheimer's disease than women. Testosterone boosts energy, too, and has a profound impact on desire and other aspects of your sex life. In addition, this hormone protects your heart, raises your confidence and sense of well-being, and a whole lot more.

I find that most of my women patients over age forty have low testosterone levels, and I consider testosterone the unsung hero of women's health. The drop in testosterone as we age takes a huge toll on women's stamina, appearance, mental acuity, general health, and happiness. Yet it is possible to change this trajectory—without a prescription. I see the results every day at my clinic, when women come to me complaining of "feeling off." Could testosterone be your ticket to looking, feeling, and functioning better? If you're over forty (or perhaps even younger), the answer is probably yes.

Most women don't know they need testosterone, and few medical professionals understand the problems associated with loss of testosterone in women. I have written *The Hormone Secret* as a wake-up call. You can achieve healthy testosterone and other hormone levels with the same strategies that work for my patients.

Don't wait till you've got hot flashes, you're stressed and exhausted, your sex life's in a ditch, and you can't sleep or focus. Don't accept weight gain and muscle loss, bone loss and memory problems. It's much easier to make small changes now.

Give Me 30 Days to Change Your Life

You don't have to resign yourself to being less than your best. We age because we lose our hormones, not the other way around. I know, because I've treated so many cases of hormone deficiency successfully. Yet *The Hormone Secret* isn't about going to the doctor. It is possible to protect the supply of testosterone (and estrogen and progesterone) your body does manufacture, utilize it more effectively, and stimulate increased production when appropriate—at home. Through healthy eating timed right, lifestyle changes, and herbs, vitamins/minerals, and supplements found in health-food and drugstores, you can look and feel younger, healthier, and happier than you have in years.

My protocols also help with weight loss and looking and feeling young *after* you've balanced your testosterone and other hormone levels. I speak regularly at medical conferences throughout the world to educate other physicians on my methods.

My 30-Day Plan is going to help you change the way you think, move, eat, and supplement—and lose eight to ten pounds while you're doing it. In the pages ahead, I will help you to:

1. Evaluate the levels of your own hormones (including testosterone) with self-tests. These self-assessments are the same ones I've used with thousands of patients. For example, you'll find the testosterone self-test on page 49. Many women discover that their scores are eye-openers. They never knew they had hormone deficiencies.

2. Heal your adrenal glands. Your adrenals manufacture testosterone and many other hormones, but stress interferes with adrenal function. When the adrenals can't do their job right, your hormone levels decline. You lose energy and have trouble managing the pressures and strains of everyday life. Adrenal fatigue, a condition symptomized by body aches, fatigue, nervousness, and sleep and digestive problems, is one of the most common and widely missed threats to our health today. My 30-Day Plan gives you step-by-step instructions for preventing and treating adrenal fatigue.

I will also show you effective ways to slash the chronic stress that stops the adrenals from producing hormones as they should. A new perspective and breathing and other exercises will focus and calm you. I will teach you how to turn off stress and turn on healing and rejuvenation. Incidentally, did you know that your body's response to stress is to produce fat? Yes, stress makes you fat.

3. Detoxify your liver. Your liver works overtime to filter all the pollution and pesticides you're exposed to. A sluggish liver performs below par. The liver also activates testosterone and other hormones and converts them into safe, cancer-protective metabolites. My detox in the 30-Day Plan (which is different from detoxification of the colon) includes a cleanse that pulls out and disposes of toxins and heals and tones the liver.

4. Eat hormone-friendly foods. Changes in what (and when) you eat will speed weight loss, boost energy, and can even help you live longer. Nutrients are the raw ingredients for building our cells, detoxifying the liver, and healing the adrenals. But our food sources are less nutrient-dense than they were fifty years ago, due to pollution, pesticides, and farming practices. I'll show you what to eat in order to compensate—and provide a maintenance guide for life after the 30-Day Plan.

5. Boost and balance hormones with herbs and supplements. My 30-Day Plan details specific herbs and vitamin/mineral supplements available over the counter to balance any hormone deficiencies you may have. For example, the herbs maca and ashwagandha help increase testosterone. Vitamin C and vitamin B complex boost estrogen levels in women.

I know my program works because I'm in the trenches all day, every day, listening to women's problems and finding solutions that will get the results everybody wants in a busy life. Often research looks good in a textbook but isn't true in clinical practice. Or, even worse, the findings are so hard to implement that patients won't follow them. Not only have I been able to prove that my plan works; I've found systems, techniques, and tricks to make research ideas doable. For example, it's fine to tell a patient, "Don't eat sugar." But the reality is that isn't going to happen in the vast majority of cases. People are far likelier to respond to: "Eat sugar twenty percent of the time if you must, and avoid it the rest of the time."

My practice is divided. I also have one of the largest nonsurgical cosmetic and skin-care practices in Seattle, where I correct what the world has done to us. My clinic is a national training center for physicians. In addition, patients are treated here for adult acne, correction of sun damage, and facial rejuvenation. I work on transformations from the inside out, but the outside affects our confidence. When you feel good, you look good; when you look good, you feel good. You have a spring in your step and feel a little happier.

It Worked for Me

I know the value of my plan, because it's changed my own life. At age forty-two, I stopped wearing skirts—my favorite things—because I had this little fat pouch at my tummy. I'd had my second child at forty-one, and gained fifty pounds with each pregnancy. My obstetrician wasn't concerned, because I am genetically on the thin side. But I was a resident and up all night every third night, and I had nausea during pregnancy. I ate normally all day, but I'd hit the cheese and crackers nonstop after the sun went down, and my stomach acted up. Boy, did I gain weight.

I did breast-feed for a year with each child, and that helped me lose the baby weight, but my body looked and felt very different. My percentage of body fat jumped 10 percent even though I weighed the same. I wasn't as patient as I wanted to be with my children. I wasn't sleeping well.

It wasn't until I balanced my own hormones—without a prescription—that my life changed. Progesterone was my biggest deficiency, and I started off with over-the-counter progesterone cream. Almost immediately, I felt calmer and started sleeping better. I had more patience with my toddlers. I also began to address my low estrogen levels, which were less problematic than my progesterone deficiency but still caused memory and focus issues. (I didn't have hot flashes, though.) I followed my own program, which did wonders for my brain.

But it wasn't until I added testosterone that I began to realize the importance of this hormone. It was my "Aha" moment. At forty-seven, I thought, "I'm doing what everyone else is doing—estrogen and progesterone—and, yes, I'm lean. But I'm not firm. I'm flabby." I knew testosterone increased the muscle-to-fat ratio, and I took two herbs that boosted my levels. Gone was the fatigue that had lingered even after estrogen and progesterone had been restored, and my sense of well-being (that hard-to-define happy place) had returned.

Let's Get Started

With the measures ahead, you can start taking control of your body, too. You can trim down fast and look younger, wake up your sex life, help your bones, heart, memory, sleep, increase strength and endurance, and so much more. No more doctor's visits to get help for fatigue and lack of energy, where you're told, "You're fine." You can become the CEO of your own health.

PART ONE

Your Hormones and the Secret Weapon

CHAPTER 1

Hormones Working Together: The Entire Orchestra

Perk up your ears and imagine sitting next to me as the curtain is about to rise on the opening night of a concert. The orchestra consists of strings, wind, and percussion sections, each tuning up with dissonant sounds. Initially, there is a kind of chaos as orchestra members practice and refine the parts they play in the performance that's about to begin. Yet slowly the instruments begin to work together in harmony. They become a cohesive unit as the curtain goes up, and the performance transports you. In many ways, your hormones, which control the functions of organs and tissues in your body, are similar to a philharmonic. Hormones must balance and work in concert with one another to create optimal health. In perimenopause or menopause, too little or too much of one hormone causes an imbalance in others and can set off a chain reaction of dysfunction. This imbalance is common, because our hormones rarely decline at exactly the same rate and pace.

That's why I often hear a familiar story when a new patient comes to my office. I always ask, "Why are you here?" The answer is usually: "I'm not really sick. But I don't have the energy I used to." Frequently, a primary-care physician has prescribed an antidepressant or sleeping pills. I point out that the symptoms of depression and insomnia are almost identical to those of hormone imbalance.

"First, let's check to see if you have any hormone deficiencies," I add. "Maybe we can restore hormone balance without adding prescription drugs that have a long list of side effects." I want to know why my patients are experiencing a problem, and address that first, rather than to simply treat symptoms.

I also explain that our years of perimenopause and menopause are associated with more significant physical changes than at any other time of life, except puberty. Loss of energy is only one of the issues. Unless an MD has taken additional education in integrative medicine or anti-aging (as I have), he/she can easily miss the very real problem of hormone imbalance. Why? Because the traditional medical education that I and other physicians received focuses on diseases and how to treat them, rather than on how to create and maintain wellness.

Hormone imbalance is not a disease, but it can wreck your quality of life. We live in a society where our hormones are depleted long before the end of our life span, and at a much earlier age than was the case for our parents or grandparents. As early as our thirties, our bodies and our hormone levels are no longer in concert. The challenge is to boost some hormones to help them recalibrate and rebalance. I'm going to educate you in how to deal with and treat any hormone deficiencies you may have. It is possible to reboot your biology with a host of nutritional and lifestyle changes, plus supplementation with herbs, vitamins, and minerals available over the counter. I help women do this every day. But first I want to help you understand the state of your own hormones.

What's Going On?

Just recently, I saw three different patients who felt desperate and didn't know what was wrong with them. One, a single high-school English teacher, was experiencing premenstrual syndrome (PMS) for the very first time at the age of thirty-nine. She complained of cramps, headaches, and other symptoms, and she felt bewildered by this new turn of events. Another patient, forty-two years old, felt guilty about how often she kept "losing her cool," after priding herself on being a patient, calm wife and mother. "This isn't me," she insisted. The third woman, forty-five, a successful business executive, was experiencing profound fatigue for no plausible reason. "I used to be a ball of energy. I don't understand what's happened to me," she said.

All three women had no idea their symptoms suggested the beginning of menopause. Neither they nor their primary-care physicians had made the connection, because they didn't have hot flashes and night sweats. Many women (and some doctors) don't associate exhaustion, irritability, brain fog, or unexplained weight gain and other menopausal symptoms with hormones. They conclude, "I'm cranky because my life is busy. I have small kids and I work. Of course I feel crappy, because I'm not sleeping. My work is stressful. I'm not losing weight, because I'm not working out." Some of these women are divorced. Some juggle a career and the care of elderly parents. Or they're stay-at-home moms, contending with stresses of their own. Whatever the individual scenario, they just accept "feeling off" as a consequence of external grievances—when it's really about internal disequilibrium that can be fixed. And the sooner the better!

What You Need to Know About Perimenopause and Menopause

People often confuse the terms "menopause," which occurs at an average age of fifty-one in North America according to the National Institutes of Health (NIH), and "perimenopause," the years leading up to cessation of your menses. Menopause simply means you have not had a period for twelve consecutive months. Perimenopause can start ten years before you hit the mark of menopause. You may experience perimenopausal symptoms as early as your thirties—and certainly your forties. Hot flashes and other symptoms are part of menopause, because they're directly related to the decline and absence of the hormones estrogen and progesterone. However, it is perimenopause that really affects your quality of life. For some women, hot flashes and night sweats start in perimenopause, the period of time when hormones begin to decline but are not yet entirely absent. Other women don't have flashes and sweats but do have mood, cognitive, weight, and other problems at this stage.

Why Is This Happening?
Your ovaries are the primary organs producing several hormones, including estrogen, progesterone, and testosterone in the childbearing years. Childbearing plays a big role in hormone levels. Pregnancy is ten months, not nine. Your ovaries and adrenal glands go into a totally different modality at this time, and hormones are different. It takes quite a while for the body to figure out how to get back to normal. For example, hair gets thick and luxurious during pregnancy. You have the same static level of estrogen and progesterone while you're pregnant. The normal cycle of your hair growing and then falling out doesn't occur. It just grows and stays.

After the baby is born, hair falls out because your hair has a lot to do with estrogen. Some women feel as if they're going crazy because they see handfuls of hair in the shower.

Not everyone has lingering hormone issues after giving birth, but a large number of women do. For nearly a year, you are pregnant and your hormones are in suspended animation They don't go through their normal rise and fall. After pregnancy our hormones rush out, and it's like pulling out a plug. There's nothing gentle about it, and it feels very abrupt. In some women, that crash in certain hormones (particularly progesterone, which drops after you give birth, sometimes causing dreadful PMS) leads to depression. It takes the body a while to "remember" and kind of grease the gears to return to its cycle.

The other problem that is common after childbirth is stress, which depletes hormones. Who is more stressed, more sleep-deprived, more exhausted than a new mom? We used to live in a village where family members, friends, and connections helped us raise a child. We don't live in a village anymore, and we lack the resources to restore our body systems by having somebody else hold the baby while we take a shower.

I remember when I was in residency and had my daughter. I'd go to the clinic early and literally lie on the floor, because I couldn't get up. I'd stay there until I had to start seeing patients. I had the physical drain of different hormones needed to produce milk, the drain of lack of sleep, and the drain of "being on call."

When I first got my pager, I was so excited. Somebody was telling me that a patient was very sick, and there were all those issues to be dealt with. I turned to the nurse and said, "You'd better call a doctor." She said, "You *are* the doctor." At that moment, I realized the responsibility I had stepped into in this long white coat. Throughout my residency, I never got over the stress of being on call.

When you're a new mom, you're on call, too. It's: "Is the baby going to cry while I shampoo my hair?" or "Will she be hungry?" And you never relax.

Maybe some new moms eat right, but I didn't. I wanted to lose the baby weight and was tired and wasn't cooking nutritious meals for myself. I didn't have to cook for the baby, who was breast-feeding. All the pillars that are the foundation for an amazing house of health—sleep, nutrition, stress management, support, relationships, doing stuff for yourself—didn't exist.

For me, it was even harder, because my husband worked out of town at the time. He was gone for three weeks and home for one week. So I was on call 24/7. He was utterly amazing when he was home, but I missed his support for our daughter and the connection we had as a family when he was away.

As you enter perimenopause, hormone production declines significantly in the ovaries, and the adrenal glands need to pick up the slack. When menstruation ceases and we enter menopause, the ovaries stop functioning and producing hormones altogether. Our bodies were designed to handle ovarian decline with the adrenal backup system to help maintain our quality of life. Today, however, the adrenals don't work well enough to produce the hormones we need. Our twenty-first-century lifestyle has created conditions that make it impossible for our adrenal glands to thrive (known as adrenal insufficiency). We're left with inadequate hormones to feel, look, and function at our best.

The Orchestra Players

As you will see, testosterone is the star of the hormone symphony. But, first, let me introduce you to the supporting cast, especially estrogen and progesterone.

Meet Estrogen

Estrogen, which is also present in men (although at a much lower level), has a big job to do for women. For example, estrogen regulates female sexual characteristics. In puberty, this hormone is responsible for the growth of curvaceous hips and full breasts. Estrogen also builds the uterine lining during the first part of a woman's menstrual cycle, in preparation for possible pregnancy. If pregnancy does not occur, this lining is sloughed off as a period.

Estrogen regulates the menstrual cycle, is in charge of the reproductive system, and supports a healthy sex life. The drop in estrogen during perimenopause and menopause plays havoc with your sexuality, causing loss of desire and vaginal dryness, which can lead to painful sex. Add night sweats and hot flashes, and it's hard to feel sexy.

Adequate estrogen levels are also essential for thinking and memory. Memory loss is a normal fact of life as the brain ages, but

> ### Optimal Estrogen Levels
>
> ❖ Help build bone
> ❖ Support your sex life
> ❖ Help your brain
> ❖ Help mood and sense of well-being
> ❖ Affect the urinary tract, heart, and blood vessels
> ❖ Support skin, hair, pelvic muscles, and breasts
> ❖ Have been shown in studies to protect against Alzheimer's disease

the loss is magnified when estrogen declines. A University of Rochester study published in 2013, in the journal *Menopause,* sheds light on the effect of menopause on cognitive functioning. Researchers followed 117 women, ages forty to sixty, in various stages of menopause and found that those who were in their first year of postmenopause experienced far greater cognitive decline and memory loss than those in perimenopause. Hormone loss was seen as the probable cause.

Estrogen and Surgical Menopause

Surgical menopause, also known as a hysterectomy (removal of the uterus) and an oophorectomy (removal of the ovaries), causes an immediate jolt to women's lives as levels of estrogen and other hormones plummet overnight. Studies show that hysterectomy shoves women into full-blown menopause earlier, even if they retain their ovaries. Depression and sexual problems, such as low libido and vaginal dryness leading to discomfort during sex, are common.

Cognition and memory often decline, too. The younger a woman is when she has surgical menopause, the faster cognition and memory issues develop, according to a study of eighteen hundred postmenopausal women. The findings were presented in March 2013 at the American Academy of Neurology.

The Estrogen Trio

There are three main types of estrogen: estradiol, estrone, and estriol. They exist in different ratios depending on the stage of life you're in.

Estradiol is the predominant hormone of our youth. In the childbearing years, our ovaries produce mostly estradiol (80 percent) and the rest is equally divided between estriol and estrone. As we enter menopause, the ratio changes, and we produce predominantly estrone. Each of these estrogens is broken down, primarily through the liver, into other estrogens, and each has a role to play in our health and the diseases that affect us.

Estrone is broken down into three different components with varying functions: 2-hydroxyestrone, 4-hydroxyestrone, or 16-hydroxyestrone. The first, 2-hydroxyestrone, helps protect us from breast cancer. In contrast, 16-hydroxyestrone helps build bone, but it encourages multiplication of cells that can cause cancer. Higher than normal levels of 16-hydroxyestrone are found in women who have breast cancer. In addition, 4-hydroxyestrone has an association with cancer, too. Fortunately, you can actually guide estrone to be more protective. I'll show you how in future chapters.

Estriol is produced in significant amounts only during pregnancy. The adrenal glands manufacture a little estriol, too. Estriol is a weaker estrogen compared with estradiol and estrone. Estriol, which is available over the counter, can alleviate hot flashes and vaginal dryness. I will discuss estriol's treatment benefits more fully in Chapter 9.

Estrogen Excess

On the other hand, too much estrogen can be a major problem as well. Studies have shown that there is a link between excess estrogen and cancer. We also know that it is not just excess estrogen but an

ESTROGEN SELF-TEST

Do You Have Low Estrogen Levels?

Major sex-hormone growth occurs during puberty and peaks at around age twenty-eight. Decline begins thereafter. Below is a list of common symptoms of estrogen deficiency.

Fill in the number at right that applies to you:

	AGREE (2)	AGREE SOMEWHAT (1)	DISAGREE (0)
1. I have hot flashes.	____	____	____
2. I have night sweats.	____	____	____
3. I have vaginal dryness.	____	____	____
4. I have bladder leakage when I cough, sneeze, or run.	____	____	____
5. I get very emotional five to seven days before my period begins.	____	____	____
6. I am over forty years old.	____	____	____
7. I have difficulty sleeping.	____	____	____
8. I have lost interest in sex.	____	____	____
9. My periods have ceased.	____	____	____
10. I have had a hysterectomy.	____	____	____

Total Score: ____

Under 4: It's unlikely that you have an estrogen deficiency.

If it's 5 or higher: It's likely that you have an estrogen deficiency.

imbalanced excess estrogen that seems to be the cause. Which age group has the highest levels of estrogen? Teenagers. Yet breast cancer is virtually unheard of until later in life, because teenage girls have all their hormones in balance, including estrogen.

Estrogen excess can occur for many reasons. Birth-control pills, which contain synthetic estrogen and progestin (synthetic progesterone), can create estrogen imbalance by raising estrogen levels. Obesity can raise estrogen levels as well. In fact, weight gain is often the first sign of too much estrogen. Estrogen makes fat, which creates more estrogen, causing more fat.

Your liver can fail to excrete excess estrogen, too. Your body is perfectly designed to use what you need and dispose of the rest, and has a system to do so. This process takes place in the liver. I'll show you how to maintain a healthy liver that does its job in Chapter 7. My liver cleanse helps ensure that all excess estrogen is eliminated.

Meet Progesterone

Progesterone is the valium that bathes the female mind and helps reduce anxiety. Remember, it is the peaceful hormone. When I had hormone trouble in my early forties, progesterone deficiency was my biggest issue. Progesterone is the culprit when women balancing work and home responsibilities experience increased frustration with the details of life, and need to exert more control to keep their cool. That's what happened to me.

Progesterone acts on the gamma-aminobutyric (GABA) receptors in the brain (the same receptors sleeping pills, anti-anxiety medication, and even alcohol act upon) to produce a calming effect that helps you sleep. GABA is the primary inhibitory transmitter in the brain, protecting our brains from damaging overstimulation. If you wake up between 2 a.m. and 4 a.m. most nights (or open your eyes in the morning more tired than you were when you went to sleep), you have a progesterone deficiency.

> ### Optimal Progesterone Levels
>
> ❖ Give you a good night's rest
> ❖ Help clear brain fog
> ❖ Help build bone
> ❖ Support normal development of neurons in the brain
> ❖ Increase libido
> ❖ Improve skin elasticity
> ❖ Have an anti-inflammatory effect
> ❖ Help prevent bloating and puffiness

Foggy Brain

Many women in perimenopause or menopause complain of "foggy brain"—and low progesterone is the troublemaker. It also causes sleep problems that worsen brain fog. Brain fog is characterized by slower processing time and difficulty finding the words you're looking for. You might be unable to retrieve the name of a coworker and have to sit down and think of it. You pull out your iPhone to make an appointment with the dentist, and find that it takes a minute to recall his name. A patient of mine, a fifty-four-year-old flight attendant, was telling a story to friends on her way to work, and couldn't retrieve the name of the Irish holiday where there's a parade and everyone dresses up in green. It took her a day to figure out that the holiday was St. Patrick's Day.

Getting Pregnant

Progesterone plays a role in embryo implantation, too. People think miscarriages and an inability to conceive are very mysterious and complicated. In medical school, I was taught that the most common reason for miscarriages is chromosomal abnormalities, and that it's nature's way of taking care of business. In fact, it turns out that miscarriages are usually caused by progesterone deficiency. When progesterone is prescribed, women are able to get pregnant and stay pregnant. It's also reassuring to know that progesterone is safe to take when you're trying to get pregnant and during pregnancy. Women who wait until their thirties to get pregnant may be surprised to learn they may have a progesterone deficiency.

Some patients are nervous about taking a hormone, and I always tell them, "Let's start with progesterone. It's the one that doesn't have any worrisome side effects, and it can have such a large impact on your life." I think progesterone is No. 2 in significance for women, after testosterone. I always say that if there's a fire in my house I would grab my children and my progesterone. My husband was a fireman, and he can run for himself.

Progesterone also affects menstruation, balances the effects of estrogen, is a natural diuretic, and helps normalize blood-sugar levels. It stimulates cells called osteoblasts, which make new bone. In our younger years, progesterone is the hormone of pregnancy. The same progesterone is focused on its function during pregnancy—"pro" meaning in favor of "gest," as in gestation (pregnancy). Progesterone is produced by the ovaries, by the placenta during pregnancy, and by the adrenal glands. After the childbearing years, it is metabolized through the liver and must be produced solely by our poor, overworked adrenal glands (along with testosterone and certain other hormones).

I know from clinical trials and from treating thousands of my own patients that progesterone levels are the earliest to decline—and they drop fast! You can have a low progesterone level as early as your late twenties. This is significant for two reasons. First, irritability, loss of enjoyment of life, and trouble sleeping are not due to stress, working hard, or getting older (though these do not help). They're caused by hormone imbalance, such as low levels of progesterone, and are easily fixed.

PROGESTERONE SELF-TEST

Do You Have Low Progesterone?

These symptoms are commonly found in women suffering from progesterone deficiency.

Fill in the number at right that applies to you:

	AGREE (2)	AGREE SOMEWHAT (1)	DISAGREE (0)
1. I have premenstrual breast tenderness.	___	___	___
2. I have premenstrual mood swings.	___	___	___
3. I have premenstrual fluid retention and weight gain.	___	___	___
4. I have premenstrual migraine headaches.	___	___	___
5. I get very emotional five to seven days before my period begins.	___	___	___
6. I have severe menstrual cramps.	___	___	___
7. I have heavy periods with clotting.	___	___	___
8. I have or have had uterine fibroids.	___	___	___
9. I have breast cysts.	___	___	___
10. I have problems with infertility.	___	___	___
11. I have had more than one miscarriage.	___	___	___
12. I have anxiety or panic attacks.	___	___	___
13. I wake up between 2 a.m. and 4 a.m. and can't get back to sleep.	___	___	___

Total Score: ___

A 6 or above indicates progesterone deficiency.

Second, when progesterone drops sooner and faster than estrogen, we become "estrogen dominant." This means that although estrogen levels are declining as well, our progesterone dips to a lower level compared with estrogen and our other hormones. This imbalance leaves us at increased risk for estrogen-related cancers.

The Testosterone Life Changer

Estrogen and progesterone are the backup players in the symphony. But testosterone is the star, because adequate levels improve almost every aspect of your health, your figure and general appearance, how you function at home and at work, and your zest for life. Sometimes testosterone is even called the personality hormone, because a healthy level actually correlates with assertiveness, motivation, and a sense of power and well-being.

Testosterone and Our Bodies

If there's a woman who's satisfied with her weight and body firmness as she gets older, I haven't met her. Yet testosterone can make an enormous and surprising difference in both. Take Mary, a thirty-nine-year-old stay-at-home mom and the wife of a construction manager. Her kids were in school, which left her time to enjoy going to the gym and playing tennis. Despite this active lifestyle and a slim body, Mary came to see me about how she could tighten her arms. She was fit, but unhappy that no matter how hard she worked on her arms she couldn't firm them up. "I've stopped wearing sleeveless tops and dresses," she told me. "I need laser treatment."

Now, my passion in life is teaching people how to boost and balance their hormones, but I am also a board-certified aesthetic physician. Blending my knowledge of cosmetic medicine with hormone medicine, I suggested, "Let's slow things down. I think I can help you get what you want without laser treatment. I'd like to try

> ### Optimal Testosterone Levels
>
> - ❖ Treat depression as well as antidepressants
> - ❖ Help you lose weight
> - ❖ Help you handle stress
> - ❖ Energize you
> - ❖ Support cognition and memory
> - ❖ Rev up your sex life, increasing desire and fulfillment
> - ❖ Keep your liver and your blood vessels clean
> - ❖ Protect your heart, body, bones, brain, and more
> - ❖ Build muscle and optimize your body's muscle-to-fat ratio
> - ❖ Improve the appearance of your skin and hair

to boost your testosterone levels instead. If I'm right, you'll save a lot of time and money."

Mary liked the idea and was willing to get her testosterone levels checked and treat her arms from the inside out. The results showed she had an active testosterone level of less than 1, when 2–5 is optimal for women. We discussed ways to boost her level. I suggested over-the-counter supplements and a topical testosterone-boosting cream. She was willing to take testosterone, but first she wanted to see if supplements worked. After sticking to her plan for four months, she was rewarded with firmer, tighter arms. Her elevated testosterone levels (without a prescription) increased the amount of muscle in her body relative to fat—and firmed the flab.

Testosterone and Life After Hysterectomy

On top of all the testosterone advantages I've already mentioned, study after study shows that testosterone is literally a lifeline for women who undergo hysterectomy. One particular research article published in 2000, in the *Journal of Women's Health & Gender-Based Medicine,* sums up the ordeal patients face. The author states that estrogen is not enough after hysterectomy, because many women also suffer undiagnosed testosterone deficiency. Symptoms of that deficiency, such as loss of libido, sexual pleasure, and a sense of well-being, go untreated. Adding testosterone to estrogen supplementation also helps prevent osteoporosis and may protect the heart.

I will spotlight testosterone exclusively in the next chapter because of this hormone's enormous significance for women—and its lack of attention from the medical community. Women have been afraid of testosterone supplementation for good reason. Years ago, the side effects of testosterone-replacement hormones were sometimes frightening, including growth of hair on the face, acne, bad temper, and other problems. We now know that these effects were due to high doses given to women. Today, the medical community agrees that women should receive only a fraction of the amount given to men.

But I'm not talking about your mother's testosterone or prescription hormones. My program is about increasing your body's testosterone naturally, on your own. I'm talking about nutrition and lifestyle changes, and supplementation using over-the-counter herbs, vitamins, and minerals.

In Chapter 2, you'll learn the incredible facts about testosterone for women and have the opportunity to evaluate your own testosterone levels with a testosterone self-test. If your levels are low—and most women's are after forty—I will explain how to increase your testosterone safely, effectively, naturally, and by yourself.

Other Parts of the Symphony

There are fifty different hormones in our bodies, but in this book I focus on a small number that have special importance for women. In addition to "the big three" (testosterone, estrogen, and progesterone), you must be aware of:

Cortisol

Cortisol is known as "the stress hormone," and nature designed it for the needs of prehistoric man, who had to fight for survival on a daily basis. If a cave man saw a big, ferocious bear, his adrenal glands responded to the perception of stress by pumping cortisol into his system, pushing him to flee this life-threatening situation. However, cortisol is very inflammatory, and its secretion was supposed to last for about two minutes, provided he wasn't eaten by the bear.

Today, big bears aren't our problem; we're exposed to different sorts of stress. Yet your adrenal glands pump cortisol in response to all perceptions of stress, including a bad day at the office or a late babysitter.

Because the adrenals are so busy with cortisol, they have less time to manufacture testosterone, estrogen, progesterone, and other hormones that make your life better and easier. When you're driving on the freeway and there's a police car behind you and sirens start blasting and lights flash, your body has a physical response. Your heart beats faster, your breathing becomes shallow, your eyes probably dilate, because you're thinking, "Oh, no! I'm going to get pulled over for speeding." This is a physical stress response caused by a cascade of stress-related hormones responding to a thought and a feeling. It is important to note how powerful a thought or feeling can be.

Stress assaults us 24/7 in our society, resulting in too much cortisol, which leads to hormone depletion. In Chapter 4, I will show you exactly how that happens. Too much cortisol due to overwhelming stress can also block progesterone receptors.

In Chapter 4, I will show you how to handle that stress in a healthy, efficient manner, and take control of cortisol overproduction.

Cortisol is also responsible for dumping sugar into the bloodstream (you need immediate energy for the fight-or-flight response). The trouble is that sugar makes our bodies produce insulin to deal with it. Insulin is secreted by the pancreas and released into the blood when glucose levels rise, such as following a meal. The insulin lowers the glucose level in the blood by transporting the glucose to the cells. When there is more glucose than the cells need at that moment, the insulin stores the excess sugar as fat. Over time the amount of insulin rises, which increases the desire and craving for more sugar in order to fill the insulin receptors. Sugar addiction has been compared to heroin addiction, due to these receptors shouting to be fed. This is one of the reasons stress causes you to gain weight and makes it almost impossible for you to lose weight. My 30-Day Plan will help you change this.

Many of my patients have elevated insulin levels and insulin resistance, a condition in which insulin becomes less effective at lowering blood sugar, which can impede weight loss. I check my patients' insulin levels to see if they are rising, as this is one of the best and earliest ways to detect prediabetes.

DHEA

DHEA is the raw ingredient of many hormones and an excellent indicator of your adrenal health. Because DHEA is a precursor to testosterone, replenishing it helps the body make more of its own natural testosterone. Studies show that the level of DHEA in your body also directly correlates with longevity. Perhaps one reason is that DHEA lowers total cholesterol and LDL (i.e., the "bad" cholesterol).

DHEA also:

1. Reverses immune suppression caused by excess cortisol levels from stress.
2. Stimulates bone production and remodeling to prevent osteoporosis.
3. Lowers LDL cholesterol (the lousy one).
4. Is important to women's libido, due to its androgen activity, and works with testosterone in this.
5. Makes more thyroid hormone available to the body.

Vitamin D

Did you know that vitamin D is a hormone, not a vitamin? It has been called the key that unlocks thousands of enzymatic reactions in your body. Vitamin D deficiency has been linked to multiple cancers, depression, and possibly even to multiple sclerosis (MS). Vitamin D is also important in the formation of bone and the prevention of osteoporosis. If you live in a latitude of 35 degrees (as I do in Seattle), you're not making enough vitamin D from October to April. You will need to supplement.

Pregnenolone

This hormone is available over the counter, and I have put some patients on it. It's one of the "mother hormones," meaning that many other hormones are made from it. In the list of hormones and what each one comes from, cholesterol is at the top and pregnenolone is next in line. I find that my healthy young patients can correct their hormone imbalances by increasing this raw ingredient.

Thyroid—the Symphony Conductor

You can't talk about the symphony without talking about the conductor. Your thyroid gland tells every cell in your body how fast or slow to go. Low thyroid hormone levels make you feel like a sloth. Everything moves slowly. You could sleep for ten hours and still feel tired. Your bowels move slowly, causing constipation, your skin becomes dry, and your hair turns coarse. Low thyroid levels can also cause an increase in cortisol production, which can make you feel wired and tired. DHEA helps convert inactive thyroid (T4) into active thyroid (T3), which makes more thyroid hormone available to the body. I'll discuss more about thyroid hormone in future chapters.

Fixing It

I'm going to show you how to stimulate your body to manufacture and balance estrogen, progesterone, testosterone, and other hormones naturally—and to make the hormones you do have as productive as possible. My mission is to empower you to take charge, to do this on your own—safely and without a visit to the doctor— and to show you why testosterone is the missing link for optimal energy and wellness.

CHAPTER 2

Is Testosterone Deficiency Making You Fat, Fatigued, and No Fun?

I f you knew about a safe, effective secret weapon for health and happiness in your life, wouldn't you use it? Adequate testosterone is that miracle worker. I find that most of my women patients lack sufficient testosterone for optimal health. Yet research shows that adequate levels of testosterone can help prevent diseases in most of our organ systems, in addition to improving our quality of life and our figures! Testosterone changes everything, protecting our heart, bones, brain, sex life, and even fighting cancer. Perhaps you've noticed that men lose more weight than women do (and lose it faster)—and seem to age more slowly and gracefully than we do as well. Maybe you've wondered why middle-aged men still want sex although we lose the intensity of our desire for it. It's because men have more testosterone than we do. And the issue is, could low testosterone be stopping you from looking, feeling, and functioning better? Hormone levels, especially testosterone levels, are rarely tested in women. But I'm going to help you take your body, brain, and health into your own hands now, just as I do for my patients. You can boost your own testosterone safely and appropriately for your age—naturally.

Listen to the experience of one of my patients, fifty-six-year-old Stephanie, an IT project manager. Stephanie, who is five-six, weighed in at 213 pounds when she walked into my clinic for her first appointment. Stephanie was a successful problem-solver who knew that she was dangerously overweight and had seriously tried to slim down on her own. She ate healthy foods most of the time. She was moderately physically active, playing golf once a week, walking for thirty minutes three times a week, and gardening on weekends. She would lose ten pounds or so, but the rest wouldn't budge, even though she'd tried Weight Watchers and other programs. Obviously, something was wrong, and I searched for more information.

Sure enough, a battery of blood tests gave me answers. Results showed that Stephanie had slight insulin resistance, a condition in which the hormone insulin becomes less effective at lowering blood sugar, which can impede weight loss. To treat the insulin resistance, I immediately removed foods from Stephanie's diet that raise blood sugar, such as sugar, fruit juices, and other simple carbohydrates. I also banned processed foods made with white flour (which quickly turns into sugar) and dairy products, which contain sugar. The ending "ose" tells us there is a sugar in the food, and when people are lactose-intolerant they can't process the sugar component in dairy products.

On the plus side, I told Stephanie to eat nutrient-dense foods like vegetables and certain fruits more often to give her body the nourishment it needed. The changes were dramatic, and they began to work quickly. Within three months, she dropped thirty-five pounds.

At that point, however, she hit a plateau, despite expanding her exercise regimen and following my food recommendations. The dial on her scale refused to drop lower. In many ways a physician is like a detective, and I ordered additional blood tests, searching for clues to why she was stuck. Test results revealed that her testosterone level was literally undetectable. One of testosterone's many functions is maintaining a healthy muscle-to-fat ratio. Muscle burns calories, and severe testosterone deficiency had slashed her body's ability to make muscle and lose pounds.

To treat Stephanie's deficiency, I put her on two products available over the counter. One was an herb that nudges the testosterone you do have (even if the amount is tiny) to be more active and available. The other product was a topical cream containing herbs that boost the body's production of testosterone. Many studies agree that testosterone reduces blood glucose to aid weight loss. Stephanie's testosterone level rose in just one month. Although her level still wasn't robust, it was high enough to kick-start a new round of weight reduction.

Symptoms of insufficient testosterone are often confused with a wide variety of conditions, including depression. The doctor prescribes an antidepressant, sends you home, and the real problem goes untreated. I'm going to help you evaluate your own signs of testosterone deficiency (if any) and provide you with the tools to take control.

The Untold Story of Testosterone

You've probably seen ads in the media about "low T" in men—and maybe you've heard that testosterone helps women's libido (sexual desire) as they age. Yet you probably don't know about the rest of testosterone's extraordinary benefits for women.

Although many studies confirm testosterone's benefits for men, less research has been available on its advantages for women, except in the area of libido and some great studies on the successful treatment of depressed women using testosterone. Many researchers have looked at estrogen, progesterone, and vitamin D, but testosterone has been overlooked. That's changing now. I'm going to educate you in the research on women that *is* available—and show you that testosterone is both safe and effective.

Testosterone Helps You Slim Down and Shape Up

Because metabolism slows as you age, it becomes harder to burn calories and maintain a healthy weight, as Stephanie discovered. Your muscle-fat ratio also changes, leaning toward fat and causing further reduction of calorie-burning power. The rise in body fat can occur even if you look thin. For example, I was a "skinny fat person." Before optimizing my testosterone, I had a higher percentage of body fat than I did years ago, although I had maintained the same weight. The reading on your scale may not show a weight change, but you may feel fat and soft. That's a red flag of low testosterone. This hormone is an important raw ingredient for muscle.

Low testosterone levels prevent your triceps curls at the gym from eliminating "waddle arm." Conversely, adequate testosterone enables you to create the ideal muscle-fat ratio. More muscle helps you lose weight and look healthier, because it burns calories even when you're at rest—while you watch TV, drive, or work on your laptop or iPad. Muscle does the work for you, which is another reason men lose more weight than women and lose it more easily. They have more muscle than we do and burn more calories sitting on the couch watching football.

In the introduction to this book, I told you about my own weight and shape issues after I gave birth to my two daughters. Boosting progesterone helped me a lot, but testosterone is the miracle worker that allowed me to create a lean, healthy body. I stimulated my body to produce more testosterone—and help the testosterone I did have to function more efficiently. How? Through changes in nutrition, use of over-the-counter herbs and supplements, special exercises, and other key changes that don't require an appointment with the doctor. You can reap the benefits, too. The best part is that when you stimulate your own testosterone production (rather than adding testosterone), you don't have to worry about an excess of this hormone.

Testosterone Zaps Osteoporosis

Another reason testosterone is a superstar hormone is that it builds bone, and does it without the scary side effects of the drug Fosamax (the most devastating of which is necrosis of the jaw). Testosterone is one of the best ways to prevent and treat osteoporosis, the condition in which bones become brittle, weakened, and prone to fracture. Throughout your life, your body goes through a process of constantly breaking down old bone and replacing it with new. As you age, however, the process lags. Less and less bone is replaced, and bones thin. Osteoporosis significantly increases your risk for breaks, especially in the wrist, spine, and hip.

Testosterone works for bone in several ways. It promotes protein synthesis and the growth of bone tissues with testosterone receptors. These receptors stimulate testosterone activity. The results we see are increased bone density and strength, and stimulation of linear growth and bone maturation. Testosterone also helps bone in another way: It can be converted into estrogen, which participates in creating strong, healthy bones. Because there are many kinds of estrogen, we want to monitor the conversion of testosterone to estrogen and ensure that it is a safe, rather than unsafe, type of estrogen. Tests help us do that. But this is a generally positive process for our bones. When testosterone and estrogen work together (in balance), their potency as bone builders is compounded.

Today, we have absolute proof that testosterone increases bone density. One of my favorite studies was published in 2006, in the *Journal of Clinical Endocrinology & Metabolism*. This study followed fifty-one women of reproductive age who were profoundly deficient in testosterone due to loss of adrenal and/or ovarian function. This twelve-month randomized, placebo-controlled, double-blind study by researchers at Massachusetts General Hospital and Harvard Medical School found that testosterone replacement increased bone density in the hips and thighs compared with a placebo.

This is a solid-gold study. The only possible criticism is that it was conducted solely on women who had profound testosterone deficiency due to loss of adrenal and/or ovarian function. In reality, all women experience a significant decrease in ovarian function as we get older, because we weren't intended to have babies in our fifties and sixties. Ovarian function declines to nearly nothing. This study would have been more meaningful if it had been conducted on all women who experienced decreases in adrenal and ovarian function.

The study used bioidentical testosterone, which mimics Mother Nature and is not synthetic. (I will discuss bioidentical hormones in detail in Chapter 11.) Researchers replaced the testosterone that had been lost to the mid-normal range—in the same amount the women's bodies were accustomed to—nothing extra. It's the little bit that we all need in order to look and function at our best.

Other research conducted exclusively on men has shown that testosterone stimulates a particular collagen bone-building activity in the body. But it really doesn't matter what sex you are, because we all have those cells. The activity mentioned in this research could be one of the reasons men are less prone to osteoporosis than we are.

Don't Be Fooled

Many of us think that osteoporosis affects other women, not ourselves. The thinking goes, "I never fall"—or "When I fell (or had my skiing accident), I didn't break anything." That's a dangerous assumption, because osteoporosis is a silent condition. You often don't know you have it until you fracture your wrist or hip. Most of my patients are surprised to learn that an osteoporosis fracture is not due to a fall. The "fall" happens because the hip fractured first. Consider the statistics:

✧ One in three women over fifty (versus one in five men) will experience a fracture caused by osteoporosis. (Compare this to women's one in eight chance of getting breast cancer during their lifetime.)

RISK FACTORS FOR OSTEOPOROSIS

The most significant risk factor is menopause—the decline of your hormones. Other risk factors include physical inactivity, smoking, alcohol, and prolonged use of corticosteroids, such as cortisone. Oddly, a high body-mass index (BMI) is actually protective against osteoporosis. This is one of the few instances where being overweight is a positive health factor.

Proton pump inhibitors, which include products like Nexium and Prilosec, are also a top risk factor for osteoporosis, because they reduce the absorption of calcium from the stomach. Lost calcium weakens bones. You'll see the warning if you read the tiny print in the directions on the acid-reflux medication package.

These drugs do eliminate acid, but the most common cause of reflux is *not* too much acid. It's food sensitivity. I challenge everyone to find out the cause of their reflux and heartburn, instead of just accepting that a proton pump inhibitor is necessary. Hundreds of my patients have resolved their acid-reflux problems by getting tested for food allergies—and simply avoiding the foods that irritate their system and thereby decreasing inflammation.

My husband has firsthand experience. Although he's of Italian descent, he's allergic to garlic. Soon after I met him, we went out to dinner. He had significant heartburn afterward, which was unusual. I suggested that he take a food-sensitivity test. The results confirmed my suspicions. He can't always avoid garlic, because sometimes it's already in the food he orders when we go out. He doesn't know about it until he has reflux that night. Many food sensitivities can be difficult to identify because you don't necessarily react right away, as you would if you ate peanuts. Sometimes, as in my husband's case, you have a delayed reaction. You might not know that your fatigue or joint pain or headache or acne or reflux is associated with the green beans you ate two days ago.

✧ Half of women who have a hip fracture never regain the quality of life they had before.

✧ In women over forty-five, osteoporosis accounts for more days spent in the hospital than other diseases, including diabetes, heart attack, and breast cancer.

✧ Just a 10 percent loss of bone can double your risk of fracture.

These statistics are more devastating than those for breast cancer, yet we're far more frightened of the latter.

The Testosterone Fat Fix

Incidentally, the same 2006 study on testosterone's bone-density powers that I mentioned earlier also showed that testosterone improves mood and body composition. Body composition was measured by the amount of body weight that was fat-free versus the amount of "fat weight." Testosterone replacement changed that balance, increasing the amount of fat-free weight, as well as thigh muscle.

A surgeon friend of mine says he can go to the beach and judge who is testosterone-deficient by the amount of fat he sees on a person's trunk after forty-five, regardless of gender. We get a layer of fat in middle age that we've never had before. Testosterone fixes that. You can do all the dieting and exercising you want after forty-five and you're not going to get the same results. Think of a rechargeable battery. Without testosterone, your battery is like one you've used for the twenty-seventh time. It doesn't completely juice up. But an adequate testosterone level makes you feel like a brand-new Duracell.

Testosterone Protects Against and Treats Depression

Women have double the risk of depression during their lifetime that men do—and 21.3 percent of us will experience a major depression.

The risk of depression seems to rise during perimenopause; in menopause, an estimated 20 percent of women are depressed. Testosterone comes to the rescue, helping women regulate their emotions and elevating mood very effectively. Testosterone also helps banish anxiety, which often accompanies depression.

In a 2012 study of depression, researchers at Florida State University found that testosterone replacement reversed depressive behavior. A specific pathway in the brain's hippocampus mediated testosterone's effects.

My patient Cheri, forty-eight, recently married for the second time, learned all about the benefits. Cheri had the life she'd always dreamed of. She and her husband had a comfortable income. Her daughter was doing well at college. She had little stress and life was good. Yet Cheri came to my office complaining of lack of interest in activities she'd previously enjoyed, along with bursts of crying spells. As we talked, she told me she'd experienced similar symptoms in her twenties, when she struggled with mild depression. But she couldn't understand her complete loss of interest in sex. She was a newlywed who loved and felt very attracted to her husband. "I've been pretty hard to live with," she admitted.

Many women share Cheri's experience. Women with a history of depression are four to nine times more likely to be depressed in perimenopause than women who haven't been depressed in the past. I started Cheri on a testosterone-stimulating herb, vitamin B complex, and an over-the-counter testosterone-boosting topical cream for women. I also recommended testosterone-friendly nutrition changes. At her three-month follow-up, she arrived smiling, and announced, "My husband wants to thank you, and so do I."

Testosterone Boosts Your Brain

Testosterone's effects on the brain have been linked to spatial relations, cognition, memory, and mood. When your brain has enough testosterone, you're more confident and less fearful. Adequate testosterone levels also improve decision-making and the speed with which you process information. Testosterone has been called the "personality hormone." Personality is always there, but, especially as we women get older, we start to rein it. We stop "leaning in." We worry about how we come across and try to justify our existence, because simply "being" isn't enough.

Testosterone allows women to use all the wisdom and experience they've accumulated in past decades—without apology. When your testosterone levels are restored to where they should be for your age group, your quality of life vastly improves. Happiness doesn't mean you skip down the street. It does mean you're happier with what looks good, smells good, and feels good in your life.

Testosterone and Dementia

In elderly men, higher testosterone was associated with better performance in tests on memory, spatial ability, and executive function in a study in the journal *Neurobiology of Aging*. In addition, there was less risk of Alzheimer's disease and increased blood flow.

Other research, in Australia, presented at the Endocrine Society's 93rd Annual Meeting in 2011, suggests that testosterone may protect women against dementia, too. Nine healthy women, ages forty-seven to sixty, who were in early menopause, received testosterone spray on their skin for a period of six months. A control group received no treatment. In the group that was treated, testosterone levels were restored to those of young women of childbearing age. Both groups took cognitive tests at the start of the study, and again at completion. At the end of twenty-six weeks, the women who were treated had improved their verbal learning and memory compared with test results at the start of the study. The control group showed no significant improvement during the same period.

This is a key finding, considering the Alzheimer's gender gap. One in six women develops Alzheimer's versus one in ten men.

Could testosterone be the reason? We have receptors in the brain that activate testosterone to do its work and protect the organ.

Testosterone Helps Your Heart

Did you know that women tend to have coronary heart disease (CHD) ten years later than men, according to the National Institutes of Health? Yet CHD (not breast cancer) is the No.1 killer of women in the United States—as well as a major cause of disability. Although heart-disease death rates have dropped in the last thirty years, they've declined less in women than in men.

Testosterone may help. Multiple studies show an inverse relationship between the degree of coronary artery disease and testosterone levels. Testosterone increases plasminogen activator inhibitor (PAI-1), which is a blood-clot buster and prevents heart attacks. A higher level of natural testosterone has been found to increase the activity of your clot busters. Many studies also agree that testosterone decreases your blood glucose, which lowers your risk for diabetes.

We do know that testosterone protects men from heart disease. It aids heart function and is associated with lower cholesterol and triglyceride levels. We also have a significant number of testosterone receptors in our heart, which protects us from cardiovascular disease. The results of a great study done on women were published in 2010, in the *Journal of the American College of Cardiology*. The researchers found that testosterone improved strength and function in postmenopausal women with congestive heart failure. Studies suggest that, after a heart attack, testosterone therapy may help remodel cardiac tissue.

Conversely, a 2010 study in the *Journal of Clinical Endocrinology & Metabolism* associates low testosterone with cardiac events in older women. A German study published in 2010, in the *European Journal of Endocrinology*, followed 2,914 women from ages eighteen to seventy-five. Researchers found that low testosterone levels were associated with an increased risk of death from any cause and with higher risk of a cardiovascular event.

New Thinking

In the past, there were concerns that higher testosterone levels caused cardiovascular disease. However, most research shows no connection between the two, according to a 2012 article in the journal *Menopause.*

Belgian research published in the June 2007 issue of the *European Journal of Endocrinology* found that higher testosterone levels may protect postmenopausal women against cardiovascular disease. The study compared sex-hormone levels in fifty-six postmenopausal women who had atherosclerosis with fifty-six controls who did not have the condition. Women who had atherosclerosis had significantly lower testosterone levels than the controls.

However, too much testosterone may increase the risk of heart disease, which is why we never want an excess.

Testosterone Lifts Your Sex Life

Sexual activity is one of the signs that your life is healthy and balanced. Yet the majority of my women patients over forty would rather read a magazine than make love. They like sex, but they don't have much desire. Does this sound familiar to you? If you have a partner you're attracted to but you don't have much desire for sex, that's a sign that your life and probably your hormones are out of balance.

Testosterone is the hormone in charge of sexual desire in men and women. In many women, low testosterone negatively affects sex drive and sexual response. According to a 2004 article in *Mayo Clinic Proceedings,* increased levels of testosterone may help women have more sexual thoughts, fantasies, activity, and satisfaction.

Women who have had a hysterectomy or an oophorectomy (removal of one or both ovaries) receive estrogen to help them make up for the sudden hormone loss, but that isn't enough for many to deal with the drop in libido, pleasure, and well-being. Research spotlighted in 2000, in the *New England Journal of Medicine,* followed seventy-five women ages thirty-one to fifty-six. The findings: A testosterone patch improved sexual function and well-being in women who had hysterectomies and oophorectomies.

Many antidepressants cause sexual side effects like low libido and anorgasmia (the inability to have an orgasm). Testosterone can help.

Testosterone Improves Skin Tone and Texture, Hair, and More

Testosterone deficiency is associated with sagging, crepey skin (including cheeks) and droopy eyes. But women who boost their testosterone notice the difference in firmer, more elastic, and toned skin. Testosterone also makes hair grow and thicken. Little girls grow pubic hair and hair under their arms due to testosterone. It's an androgenic activity. As we get older and lose testosterone, our hair becomes drier and thinner. That's why so many older women have "bald spots" in the back of their heads.

Our lips thin as we age, too, due to bone loss in the upper jaw. Testosterone helps on two levels. It helps keep that bone. In addition, the lips are a muscle that atrophies with age, and testosterone builds muscle to reduce thinning.

Testosterone Fights Cancer

We tend to think that cancer is something we "get." Yet the fact is that we all have cancer cells in our bodies. Cancer is uncontrolled growth of cells. Usually, dysfunctional cells are killed by other cells to keep the body running smoothly. There is also a programmed death process called apoptosis, which kills cells that have outlived their functional life before they start becoming dysfunctional and causing problems.

Cancer cells evade this programmed death. They spread past their normal boundaries and grow faster than usual. That's how we find cancer. When a patient is diagnosed with breast cancer, her/his physician does a PET scan (positron-emission tomography) to see if the cancer has spread to other places. The scan looks for highly active cells, which I compare to a three-year-old on too much sugar. Cancer cells bounce around like cells with ADD. These agitated cells consume a lot of energy, too, which is why cancer patients become wasted.

Research suggests that testosterone is super-helpful in preventing the spread of cancer. A Swedish study published in 2007, in *Menopause,* the journal of the North American Menopause Society, is the first randomized, prospective, double-blind study of breast-cell proliferation in women. ("Proliferation" is the term for cells gone crazy, rapidly dividing and moving beyond boundaries, like breast cells growing into tumors or migrating to the brain or the bones.) This study meets all the criteria for rock-solid research. How many women were involved? Ninety-nine, which is pretty good. How did they check the breast cells? By biopsy, rather than by reading a mammogram, where results could be subject to interpretation. The first group received estrogen and a testosterone patch for six months. The control group received estrogen and a placebo patch. Results: The placebo group had more than a fivefold increase in total breast-cell proliferation. In contrast, the estrogen-plus-testosterone group had no increase in proliferation.

That means if you're taking estrogen for hot flashes and your doctor is wise enough to give you progesterone you really need testosterone as well if you want breast-cancer protection. Lots of women who have had breast cancer, or had the BRCA gene, and had their ovaries removed (surgical menopause) to prevent more cancer have hot flashes and do start estrogen. But these patients are left wondering if the estrogen will induce breast cancer.

Why aren't these women being given testosterone? It's just the evolution of medicine. When I was starting out, we gave women calcium to prevent osteoporosis and paid no attention to vitamin D. Now vitamin D is the mainstay of osteoporosis treatment. A low vitamin D level puts you at risk for osteoporosis, which is one of the reasons to get a bone scan. We didn't know what we didn't know.

Another study, by the Federation of American Society for Experimental Biology (FASEB), in 2000, looked at the effects of progesterone, estrogen, and testosterone on breast-cell proliferation in primates (rhesus monkeys). Estrogen caused a roughly sixfold increase in mammary cells. Progesterone had no effect on the cells. But testosterone slashed estrogen's breast-cell proliferation by about 40 percent. The researchers concluded that combining estrogen and testosterone can reduce the risk of breast cancer associated with estrogen replacement.

Bioidentical estrogen replacement increases proliferation, and that's why we think estrogen alone is bad for breasts and why we must respect the symphony of hormones. We know that progesterone does help modify the proliferation. But in this study the testosterone decreased the proliferation and entirely abolished the estrogen-induced receptor expression. Women have to take tamoxifen when cancer is fed by estrogen—but testosterone erased that.

We're so fearful of testosterone when we should probably be fearful of *not* having testosterone. Unfortunately, large doses given to women in the past ruined everything and scared them to death, due to side effects like hair growth on the face and acne. Overly high dosages can be common in brand-new medicines. When birth-control pills were first introduced, the doses were much higher than they are now. The same thing happened with HIV medication. Initially, big doses were used. In the first AZT trials, we learned that much lower dosages could be effective.

Safe, Effective Testosterone Treatment When Needed

Some women need more help than nonprescription testosterone boosting. Why? For a combination of reasons. If you have a huge deficiency, you may need more than your adrenal glands can produce, even with all the help I've laid out. If you've had a hysterectomy, your hormone levels have been slashed overnight. In addition, we're not all the same. Some women's "normal" level (i.e., their level at age twenty-three) may have been much higher than the levels of other women. Even if their level is measured at age fifty-three and it's in the normal range, it may represent a 75 percent decline from that in their twenties. That's a huge drop. Maybe their body didn't read the textbooks, and their normal is quite high.

For women who require it, there is low-dose bioidentical testosterone replacement. Bioidentical hormones mimic the body's own hormones and are available through compounding pharmacies, which customize medications to fit the needs of individual patients. However, I'm not suggesting that women pump their bodies full of testosterone. Low dosage is the key. I prescribe 1–5 mg when necessary, providing only as much testosterone as is appropriate for a patient's age. A small amount vastly increases a woman's quality of life. A report in the May 2012 issue of *Menopausal Medicine*, a journal of the American Society for Reproductive Medicine, emphasizes that only dosages appropriate for women should be used when testosterone is prescribed for female patients.

I start with 1 or 2 mg and slowly raise the dose, providing only as much testosterone as has been lost. At my clinic, I find that side effects in women receiving these low doses are extremely rare. In the small percentage of women who do experience problems, these effects disappear as soon as testosterone is stopped—and they do not return.

Another concern expressed at times is that no studies have been done on long-term testosterone use in women—only in men. However, the medical community has always considered results of research on males to be applicable to women as well. In addition, there

DO YOU HAVE LOW TESTOSTERONE?

Evaluate your own testosterone levels. Many women discover that their scores are eye-openers. Below is a list of symptoms most commonly found in women suffering from testosterone deficiency.

Fill in the number at right that applies to you:

	AGREE (2)	AGREE SOMEWHAT (1)	DISAGREE (0)
1. My sex drive has decreased.	____	____	____
2. I lack the drive or assertiveness I once had.	____	____	____
3. My self-confidence has declined and I feel more hesitant.	____	____	____
4. I feel constantly fatigued.	____	____	____
5. I tire easily during and after physical activity.	____	____	____
6. I have lost muscle mass, strength, or tone.	____	____	____
7. I have gained body fat around my waist.	____	____	____
8. I have elevated cholesterol.	____	____	____
9. I experience unexplainable unhappiness.	____	____	____
10. I have been diagnosed with osteoporosis or osteopenia.	____	____	____

Total Score: ____

Over 4 indicates low testosterone.

are a number of good studies that show the safety of testosterone use for women, such as the 2012 report in the journal *Menopausal Medicine*. It found no evidence that past users of testosterone have an increased risk of breast cancer or that the duration of testosterone use increases the risk of breast cancer.

Is Testosterone Loss a Problem for You?

Testosterone is called the hormone of the life force. It creates more energy because it makes life so much easier for you. Few people understand that testosterone is necessary to living a healthy and happy life—or know about the myriad problems associated with the loss of testosterone in women. Before menopause, testosterone levels drop 50 percent from levels at age twenty. Low levels correlate with depression, osteoporosis, rise in body fat, and other unwanted developments. Could testosterone be your missing link to looking, feeling, and functioning better? You may be surprised. The majority of women in their forties, fifties, and beyond have low testosterone. Luckily, we can change that!

CHAPTER 3

Boost/Balance Testosterone and Other Hormones Naturally

I didn't write this book to tell you to see a physician and get a prescription for hormone-replacement therapy. You don't have to consult an anti-aging doctor to help boost or balance your levels of testosterone and other necessary hormones. There's a lot you can do on your own to give your body what it needs to create health. In this chapter, I'm going to help you understand how to eat differently and deliciously and take other measures to protect and raise testosterone and other essential hormone levels. For example, specific herbs, vitamins, and minerals that are available over the counter can help you achieve your goals. These natural substances keep your hormones working in harmony and relieve various symptoms of deficiency.

What It Means to Boost and Balance

When I talk about boosting and balancing hormones, the task is to increase hormone levels in some cases and lower them in others, or a combination of the two. However, if you're over forty-five you probably need a boost for most of your hormones. You can stimulate your body to produce higher levels. In certain instances, you can actually increase the amount of *hormone activity* without increasing the amount of the hormone. This is accomplished in two ways—by (1) converting an inactive form of a hormone (which doesn't do the job the hormone should) into an active form that works; or (2) by kicking a hormone off its carrier protein. Some of our testosterone (and estrogen, too) is bound to a carrier protein that prevents it from reaching its receptor elsewhere in the body and becoming activated to do its job.

Here is a brief introduction to each of the important hormones that affect your quality of life pre-, during, and postmenopause—and the issues that reduce their production and performance. You'll learn how to use each of them to create a better body, brain, and life with my 30-Day Plan later on.

Testosterone

I begin with the dietary segment of boosting and balancing, because the foods you eat play such a vital role in hormone health. For example, my patients know the meaning of the word "nutrient," but most have never heard of the term "micronutrient." When I mention the word, the usual response is "What's that?" If you have a similar reaction, you're about to fill this gap in your education. Micronutrients in your diet are substances that enable your body to produce testosterone and other hormones. They are vitamins and minerals that are found in the foods we eat. But I am going to focus on plant-based micronutrients, specifically fruits and vegetables. Micronutrients are also the materials used to create the cells of the body (including organs and hormones). Micronutrients are vital to our health, longevity, and the quality of day-to-day life.

On the other hand, macronutrients (which include protein, fat, and carbohydrates) provide the energy to do that work. In the Western world, we consume more macronutrients than we need, and the body stores the excess energy as fat. We eat far too few micronutrients, which shortchanges us of the ingredients to make perfect cells. Insufficient micronutrients may be an important aspect of cancer. Although supplements can be a great way to improve micronutrient content in your diet, the very best way to get micronutrients is from food.

Testosterone-Friendly Foods: The Hidden Sugar in Your Diet

How do you maximize testosterone-friendly nutrition? You cut out sugar and saturated fats like pizza, dairy products, hamburgers, and processed meats such as bacon and sausage. Instead, you pile your plate with veggies and fruits. A patient of mine is fond of saying, "Sugar is my enemy." And she's so right. Sugar, specifically, has been shown to be a leading factor in low testosterone. Testosterone levels drop after you eat sugar, probably because it leads to a high insulin level. Your body pumps more insulin to cope with sugary foods, which triggers a cascade of reactions that reduce testosterone. Yet the average American consumes twelve teaspoons of sugar a day, which adds up to roughly two tons of sugar in a lifetime.

We love sugar because the sweet taste is pleasurable. When sugar hits your tongue, nerve impulses cause the release of opiates, a similar but weaker version of heroin or morphine. That's what keeps us coming back for more (and more) cake and ice cream and chocolate. By reducing or eliminating the sugar you eat (other than sugar found in real food, like apples), you lose weight and decrease your cravings. Sugar receptors down-regulate due to disuse. And that's just the beginning. When you peel off pounds, you also lose body fat, improve your muscle-fat ratio, and burn calories without any extra effort. It's a win-win all around.

Celebrity nutritionist, fitness expert, and *New York Times* bestselling author JJ Virgin says that most of her clients are confused by sugar, controlled by sugar, or both. JJ points out that people don't realize how much sugar they're actually consuming because they're not eating donuts or putting sugar in coffee. What they don't understand is that other foods, which seem to be healthy options, can have an enormous sugar impact. For example, yogurt with fruit is not as healthy as you think. The fructose (sugar found in fruit) has a high sugar impact on your body.

Lowering sugar means weight loss, and the extra benefit of fewer pounds for your testosterone level is that fat loss decreases the activity of an enzyme called aromatase. Aromatase is produced by your fat. (Yes, fat is an organ that produces stuff.) Aromatase takes your testosterone and converts it into bad (i.e., cancer-causing) estrogen. Less testosterone becomes available to your body. Studies show that losing weight directly increases your testosterone levels, which, in turn, increases your ability to make muscle instead of fat.

Sugar and the Glycemic Index of Food

The problem is not so much the amount of sugar your body has to handle; it's the hit of sugar that must be dealt with all at once. High-glycemic-index foods (GI) are absorbed and turned into sugar fast. They raise your blood-sugar levels quickly and stay elevated for too long. Many of these foods are not the ones you'd normally associate with sugar. For example, who doesn't love bagels? But we don't connect bagels with sweet taste. Bagels have little or no protein or fiber, although they do have plenty of calories—and a glycemic index of 72. The glycemic index of a doughnut is 76.

I regularly see how hidden high-GI foods can hijack women's weight loss, as my patient Molly found out. Molly, thirty-six, came to me to increase her energy and help her break free of her unsuccessful slimming efforts. We balanced her hormones, including boosting her testosterone, using the program outlined in this book. She also focused on her nutrition and began to work out four days a week. Molly's weight loss was more than just about looking her best. Her blood tests showed that she had met most of the criteria to be given a diagnosis of diabetes.

Molly spent six months successfully losing weight, but her blood-sugar tests showed continuously elevated levels. Only when I asked her to tell me everything she ate in a three-day period did I discover that, although she wasn't eating "junk," she was making high-glycemic choices throughout the day, including mashed potatoes and rice crackers. A quick review of the GI of foods, and the goal of eating only foods with a GI of 50 or less, paid off for Molly. Within three months, her blood tests revealed that she was no longer diabetic.

When you eat a high-glycemic food, your body experiences a sugar spike and a surge of insulin and doesn't know what to do with it. It can't use all that energy (sugar is energy) all at once, and stores the excess as fat. The same thing happens when you eat white bread, pasta, and even whole wheat bread (GI 70).

In order to lose weight and maximize testosterone, most of what you eat should be foods with a glycemic index of 50 or lower. However, even some fruits are high in sugar. For example, eat a chunk of watermelon and you may as well swallow a spoonful of sugar. The glycemic index for watermelon is in the nineties. (Remember, the goal is to stick to 50 or less.) Kids love tropical fruits. But what about the sugar in pineapple and mango? Does that mean you can never eat a bagel or a watermelon? No, but eat them sparingly and put them in the category of a treat.

Foods such as processed cereals, white potatoes, dried fruit, and pumpkin are also high-glycemic. Pasta turns into sugar immediately, and is high-glycemic. Your body has to deal with the hit all at once.

Fortunately, there are several free apps about the glycemic index that may help you identify and avoid high-GI foods. Or you can check out the foods you eat most often on any one of hundreds of free glycemic-index charts on the Web, including my website, drtami.com.

The Roles of Protein and Fats

Another way to boost testosterone is to increase the protein in your diet, because protein builds muscle. Protein takes the edge off hunger, too. But it has to be the right kind of protein. A thick, juicy steak is full of protein, but it's also loaded with bad fat. We have, however, found that grass-fed beef has a lot less bad fat than regular beef. In Chapter 6, I'll show you how protein eaten in the morning can stabilize blood sugar and curb calorie consumption effortlessly.

We also need "good fat," such as olive oil and avocado. We have a nonfat focus in our diet, but we've never been fatter, because we eat the wrong kind, such as the saturated fats in mayonnaise, margarine, whole milk, and cheese. Or, worse, we try to eat no fat. We need fat. I'll show you why and explain the skinny on fat later on.

Help from Herbs and Vitamins/Minerals

Nutrition changes provide the best environment for your body's production of testosterone. But they aren't the only tools in your arsenal. Herbs, vitamins, minerals, and other over-the-counter products can help stimulate your own testosterone production—or raise the amount of testosterone activity. To illustrate the latter, I tell my patients to visualize a band on a bus going to play a gig. In order for the band to perform, it must first board the bus. The band must then get off the bus and enter the auditorium. Testosterone is the band. The bus is the carrier protein that testosterone is bound to. The receptor is the concert hall. Testosterone has to reach the receptor in order to become active and function properly. As we get older, we have less unbound, or free, testosterone available to our body—and the remaining inactive testosterone is stuck on the bus. As a result, there is no concert. Testosterone can't do its job. This is one important reason that, if you get your blood levels tested, you need the test for free testosterone, not total testosterone. I will discuss blood tests in Chapter 12.

Following are the herbs, vitamins, and minerals that increase testosterone in women who have scored low on the testosterone self-test in Chapter 2. I will tell you exactly how much of each to use (and for how long).

Caveat: Herbs, vitamins/minerals, and other supplements can have interactions with various medications. Before taking any of these recommendations, consult your doctor to ensure that they are safe in combination with your meds (if any). Realize that anything that's powerful enough to do good is also powerful enough to do harm.

Herbs

- **Ashwagandha.** This is an ancient herb that raises testosterone levels mainly by helping the adrenal glands, which manufacture testosterone. Ashwagandha rejuvenates the adrenals and is anti-inflammatory and very important for strength. It is called an adaptogen, a nontoxic substance that helps the body reduce damage from stress.
- **Maca.** This plant, part of the broccoli family, is grown only in Peru. Maca does not increase total testosterone levels. But it does help increase the amount of active testosterone, because it kicks the hormone off the carrier protein that prevents activity and makes it more available for your body to use.
- **Mucuna Pruriens.** This Ayurvedic herb has been used for centuries to increase libido and energy, optimize blood sugar, and improve mood. It's also an adaptogen, which stimulates the cells when needed and calms when needed. It's not a depressant, so you won't get a hangover. It's not a booster, so you don't have to worry about feeling aggressive and charged up. It's been shown to improve the neurotransmitter dopamine, too, which is necessary for optimal brain health. Dopamine helps you get out of bed in the morning and take charge of your day. It controls the hormone center of the brain. Mucuna pruriens is also a

growth-hormone booster and reduces levels of prolactin (which decreases levels of testosterone).

✧ **Stinging-Nettle Root.** This herb supports free levels of testosterone and dihydrotestosterone (DHT), which is the stronger version of testosterone, by unbinding it from the binding globulins. Some people make more DHT than testosterone; it's part of the testosterone family, just as there are three different types of estrogen.

✧ **Tribulus.** This herb, which is also known as "puncture vine," has been used for some sexual problems and to improve athletic performance. Tribulus has clinically been shown to increase testosterone levels, but not when used alone. It appears to provide additional support to our bodies' own production of testosterone when used with other supplements.

Vitamins/Minerals

✧ **Vitamin B Complex.** This is especially helpful in boosting testosterone.

✧ **Vitamin C.** Helps increase testosterone levels.

✧ **Vitamin D.** Appears to have a correlation with testosterone. If you have a low vitamin D level, you may also have low testosterone.

✧ **Zinc.** This mineral is a great way to boost testosterone, because it blocks the activity of the enzyme aromatase, which transforms testosterone into estrogen. Zinc is also needed for the adrenal glands, the testosterone-manufacturing factory after age forty. Zinc accelerates the renewal of skin and hair cells, too. Zinc is so good for skin, it's a central part of the acne program at my clinic.

Our diet is very low in zinc, especially if you're a vegetarian, because we think chemicals used in conventional farming methods deplete the soil of nutrients, and nutrients like zinc must be absorbed by a plant in order for you to receive its benefits. If you take just zinc as a supplement, be careful that you don't create another deficiency in copper, as they compete with each other. For every 30 mg of zinc, you need 2 mg of copper.

You can get zinc from a multivitamin, but it is also available from food sources like beans, yogurt, kefir, raw milk, and raw cheese. According to a study published in the *Journal of Nutrition* in 1996, zinc deficiency lowers testosterone levels.

✧ **DHEA.** This hormone supplement is available over the counter. DHEA is made by the adrenal glands and is the raw ingredient for many hormones, but especially testosterone. When the adrenal glands are overworked, DHEA production is one of the things they feel they don't really need to do. Our DHEA levels drop naturally at age thirty, so some women need help getting more of this hormone.

Lifestyle

Sleep Factor

I know that most of us would like to take a few vitamins and have all our hormone imbalances restored and optimized. Unfortunately, our bodies are amazing, complex systems that need more than a quick fix. Our bodies have chemistry (the hormones and other things we can measure with a blood test and treat with medication and vitamins). Our brains and hearts operate electrically, and we view their functions by looking at their electric currents. Last, our bodies embrace what can best be described as spiritual forces. No matter what your belief or religion, how you feel affects your health. It's not surprising that we need to address more than just chemistry in order to optimize and balance our hormones.

Which brings us to the subject of sleep. Sleep is a key spoke on the wheel of optimal health, and is often affected by hormone imbalances. Women who have had no sleep issues at all may start waking between 2 a.m. and 4 a.m. in their late forties and fifties. Sleep problems affect 40 percent to 50 percent of women going through perimenopause and menopause—and can reduce levels of testosterone (and estrogen).

Do you have trouble falling asleep, turning from side to side in a futile attempt to find a comfortable position? Or is interrupted sleep a problem? Do you regularly wake in the middle of the night and find it difficult or impossible to doze off again? Or maybe you wake in the morning feeling tired and sluggish instead of refueled? For most women, these issues go hand in hand with the menopausal years. Symptoms like hot flashes and night sweats are part of what keeps us awake. But if you don't have these symptoms you may still have sleep problems caused by hormones.

The effects of lack of sleep can be downright scary, causing difficulties with memory, problem-solving, and ability-to-learn issues. New research published in the *European Heart Journal* in 2013 links insomnia with an increased risk of heart disease. The study of 54,279 Norwegian adults found that subjects with one symptom of insomnia had a 17 percent increased risk of heart disease. Two symptoms correlated with a 92 percent increase. Subjects with three symptoms of insomnia had a 353 percent increased risk of heart disease.

Research also suggests a link between the drop in sleep duration for Americans in recent years and the rise in obesity. We're sleeping less, and we're fatter than ever. A 2006 Nurses' Health Study followed a group of women for sixteen years. The authors found an association between short sleep duration and weight gain. If you sleep less than seven hours a night, you may be able to prevent obesity by increasing sleep time.

The Facts About Sleeping Pills Many of us turn to prescription sleeping pills for help when we can't sleep. It's estimated that anywhere from 4 percent to 10 percent of American adults (mostly women) use prescription sleeping pills. And research here and abroad suggests that the numbers are rising. Medications used to induce sleep include benzodiazepines, antidepressants, and antihistamines. Zolpidem (Ambien) is in a category all its own. Zolpidem works by mimicking GABA, the neurotransmitter that calms down excitement and agitation. GABA gives us the feeling of just having had a massage or relaxing in a spa.

Many sleeping pills (including Ambien) prevent REM sleep in some people. REM sleep is one of the five stages of sleep that make us feel we've had a restorative night's rest. Often, sleeping pills put you to sleep for eight hours, but you may wake up feeling sluggish.

In January 2013, the FDA reduced the recommended dose of zolpidem for women because many of them were waking with active levels of the drug in the blood—leading to drowsiness, driving accidents, and other serious consequences. Men are affected, too, but to a lesser degree than women, because women metabolize Ambien differently.

This issue is particularly important because women have been prescribed doses of Ambien twice as high as necessary for the last twenty years. The FDA recommends that dosages of regular Ambien for women be cut from 10 mg to 5 mg, and to 6.25 mg from 12.5 mg for the extended-release version. Why? Because 15 percent of women on 10 mg of Ambien are cognitively impaired at that dosage in the morning.

The results of a study published in 2012 highlights another cause for concern. Researchers examined the electronic medical records for 10,529 patients (mean age fifty-four) who took hypnotic prescription drugs (sleeping pills)—and 23,676 controls—for two and a half years. Those who took sleeping pills had triple the increased risk of death of women who did not. This was true even when the women took fewer than eighteen pills a year. The top one-third heaviest users of sleeping pills had an increased risk of developing cancer.

There are several natural ways to help with sleep. Melatonin, "the sleep hormone," is just one nonprescription option. Melatonin is made in the pineal gland, a tiny gland in the center of our brain.

Melatonin is made from tryptophan, which is also used to make serotonin (the feel-good hormone) by using vitamin B, and is a powerful antioxidant with possible anti-cancer effects.

Melatonin is produced in darkness. Even minimal light from the clock, cell phone, or iPad plugged in at your bedside interferes with your body's melatonin production. Melatonin is available over the counter and can help. However, it works best when you sleep in a pitch-black room. A review of studies in the Medline database (1975 to March 2003) confirms the benefits of melatonin, and I can tell you from my patients' experiences that it works without the impairment in cognitive function and other side effects of prescription sleeping pills. I will provide instructions on how to determine your own individual dosage of melatonin in Chapter 10. Progesterone cream, available over the counter, can also help improve sleep.

Exercise Wisely

We used to think you had to engage in high-intensity exercise to increase testosterone. But recent studies of mice show that exercise can boost your testosterone levels—and it's not the extreme exercises you'd expect. It's moderate activity, like walking.

Walking for thirty minutes five days a week is one of the best ways to exercise. You don't have to become a marathon runner. You just have to find an activity you like. Normal people like me don't have to join a gym to lift weights or sweat buckets in a spin class (unless you love that). I just go for a walk, and I feel fantastic. Exercise is good for your sex life, too. Working out increases endorphins, calms you down, and helps you look (and therefore feel) better about yourself.

If you take an antidepressant, you may know that these meds can reduce sexual arousal. Results of research in the *Annals of Behavioral Medicine,* in 2012, found exercise changed that, enhancing general sexual arousal in women taking antidepressants. The biggest improvement occurred in women who had the lowest arousal to begin with. In addition to the benefit to testosterone and other hormone levels, exercise has repeatedly been shown to be more effective than medication as a treatment for depression—and without side effects!

In Chapter 4, I discuss how powerful breathing exercises, tai chi, meditation, and other practices make you feel strong and alive and directly affect your hormone levels.

Reduce Stress

Erasing stress is another way to boost testosterone. Testosterone is manufactured in your adrenal glands, but stress upsets the adrenals' production schedule. The adrenals become so busy pumping out the stress hormone cortisol that they don't have time to make testosterone (or estrogen and progesterone). The exercises I just mentioned help here, too, and are among the tools that allow you to cope with stress effectively.

Stress also works in conflict with our hormones. When you're chronically stressed, even mildly, your body's slow but constant production of cortisol works in opposition to testosterone. Cortisol is catabolic (which means that it breaks tissue down). In contrast, testosterone is anabolic (builds up bone and muscle).

Keeping your body healthy enables it to produce your own testosterone and to utilize the testosterone you already have—completely safely.

Estrogen

As women get older, many of us become estrogen-dominant. We have a relative excess of estrogen and too little or no progesterone. These hormones are meant to work together. You don't want to isolate one hormone and treat it alone—that causes an imbalance. Some of us experience hot flashes and night sweats early, which can indicate early estrogen loss. For other women, the symptoms appear late. We are all women, but we are all individuals. The hormone self-test on page 21 will help you identify what is going on in your own body and life.

We want to encourage estrogen-like activity and boost estrogen naturally.

Estrogen-Friendly Foods

One way to reap the benefits of estrogen is to become aware of foods (called phytoestrogens) that contain estrogen or have estrogen-like activity—and increase your consumption of those. These foods include legumes, such as beans, peas, and lentils, which are high in fiber and protein yet low in fat. Soybeans, especially, contain isoflavonoids, which are a type of phytoestrogen ("phyto" meaning plant-based). Eating legumes is great because they're not going to boost your estrogen; they're going to act like estrogen and help balance hormones.

Bran, beans, fruits, vegetables, and flaxseeds contain another type of phytoestrogen called lignans. Flaxseeds are the lignan champions. They contain seventy-five to eight hundred times more lignans than other plant foods. To make your life easy, I want you to know how to use them. Buy flaxseeds in any health-food store. Sprinkle them in yogurt. Put them in your cereal. Soak them first and throw them in your smoothie to blend perfectly. I grind up flaxseed in my little coffee grinder and add a tablespoon to my pancake mix, muffin mix, and my chocolate chip cookies. Look for the really great blue-corn tortilla chips, which are infused with flaxseed.

Peas and pinto and lima beans contain yet another type of phytoestrogen—coumestan. Coumestans bind to estrogen receptors and give you the benefits of estrogen without actually having more estrogen.

Vitamin C, carotene, and B-complex vitamins are useful in raising estrogen levels (mostly in the way they help your adrenals). Whole grains can also be helpful. Be aware, however, that you can be fooled by marketing. Whole wheat is not a whole grain, although it's marketed to make you think it's healthy for you. If the words "whole wheat" do not appear first or second in the package's ingredients list, the product can have as little as 1 percent of what is being advertised.

Soy has an estrogen-like property and is great for estrogen activity—but not all soy is created equal. There is ongoing research about the safety and efficacy of isolated soy isoflavone supplements. I currently advise using natural soy foods instead. Even then, you have to be careful, because sometimes soy is not considered a food product and is not subject to FDA safety regulations. Soy is often imported from China, where standards for contamination and consistency are far below our food-safety standards.

Sprouts, cherries, apples, pomegranates, papaya, and plums are good for boosting estrogen levels. So are barley, hops, oats and brown rice, eggplants, celery, tomatoes, yams, clover, garlic, licorice, parsley, and sage. Rosemary deserves a special mention, because it converts bad (cancer-causing) estrogen into good estrogen.

The form of estrogen known as 16-hydroxyestrone is pro-carcinogenic and can actually promote breast-cancer cell formation. You can help change that effect by eating cruciferous veggies like broccoli, in addition to rosemary. On the other hand, if you have too little of 16-hydroxyestrone your bones suffer. And overdosing on cruciferous vegetables can affect your thyroid. You have to be careful. Luckily, most people don't chow down on Brussels sprouts every day.

Nobody knows the exact amount of these foods you should eat, but consciously, mindfully increase your consumption of them if your score on the estrogen self-test on page 21 shows you are low in estrogen. For example, I love fennel, but in the past I often forgot about it. I choose to eat a lot more now. I also love sunflower seeds, but, unless I make a point of paying attention, I hardly ever eat them. The same is true of cherries, except in summer. Even I forget to purposely include these foods in my diet. I have to be very mindful, physically add them to my shopping list, and have them in my home on a regular basis. Because of this, I actually planted fennel for the first time in my garden. Little did I know that fennel is easy to grow, which is a requirement for me.

I encouraged a patient, who has a condo apartment in downtown Seattle, to start a garden. She said she had a tiny patio deck only. Being creative, she bought a trellis and mounted it on the side wall of the deck and attached pots to it. She now has a wall of pots of vegetables and herbs and makes fresh, homemade salad from her patio. No weeding!

Help from Herbs and Vitamins/ Minerals for Estrogen Balance

Balancing estrogen is not a matter of increasing estrogen levels only—it's more complicated than that. I recommend the following to my patients for a variety of reasons:

✧ **Chasteberry.** This herb raises progesterone levels, which has a rebalancing effect when you've got too much estrogen (estrogen dominance). Be careful about taking this if you're taking drugs to treat psychotic disorders or Parkinson's disease, or metoclopramide because of undesirable interactions with estrogen.

✧ **Dong Quai.** This is a Chinese herb that is now made in the United States. It's traditionally been used to treat menstrual problems. Caution: It can interact with blood-thinning medications like warfarin.

✧ **Red Clover.** This prairie herb is native to Europe. It contains phytoestrogen and isoflavon estrogen-like compounds and can stimulate estrogen production.

- **Black Cohosh.** Traditionally used to treat hot flashes. It doesn't have any estrogenic activity, but it has been shown to help with symptoms that are associated with estrogen deficiency.
- **Boron.** May increase estrogen levels and reduce vaginal discomfort associated with sex after menopause. It may also have cognitive benefits.
- **Vitamin A.** A South African study found that vitamin A increased estrogen in women with menorrhagia (excessive menstrual bleeding or prolonged flow).
- **Vitamin B6:** A 1983 double-blind study reported in the *Journal of Reproductive Medicine* (regarding the etiology of premenstrual tension) found that the administration of B6 vitamins reduces the amount of estrogen found in the blood and increases progesterone, creating more balanced estrogen.
- **Vitamin C.** This is useful in raising estrogen levels.
- **Carotene.** Helps boost estrogen.
- **Vitamin E.** May be helpful for hot flashes and reducing vaginal dryness. Low levels of vitamin E are associated with estrogen deficiency.
- **Zinc.** Prevents excess estrogen.

There are also some foods that are rich in vitamins that help the adrenal glands produce more estrogen. For example, foods rich in vitamin C include kiwis, tomatoes, oranges, cantaloupes, peaches, bananas, artichokes, asparagus, carrots, cauliflower, corn, and lima beans. Carotene-rich foods include peppers, kale, spinach, carrots, beets, dandelion greens, turnip greens, cabbage, pumpkins, chard, collards, basil, and squash. Throw them in your smoothies for an awesome health boost. And don't forget beets, tuna, oats, turkey, bananas, Brazil nuts, potatoes, avocados, and legumes, which are all full of vitamin B complex.

Too much or too little estrogen can cause moodiness, breast tenderness, bloating, and sedation. Multiple studies have shown the link between estrogen dominance and some cancers. Estrogen must be balanced by the right amounts of progesterone and testosterone.

Lifestyle

Changes in lifestyle can also help balance estrogen. The results of a University of Minnesota study, published in 2013 in *Cancer Epidemiology, Biomarkers & Prevention*, found that aerobic exercise led to alterations in estrogen metabolism that may prevent breast cancer.

Too Much of a Good Thing—Reducing Estrogen

If you have ovarian or breast cysts or fibroids, they could be exacerbated by estrogen-friendly foods. Foods that inhibit estrogen production include melons, pineapples, berries, figs, grapes, green beans, corn, broccoli, white rice, and white flour. Avoid foods, like soy, that have estrogen-like activity and foods that boost estrogen.

A Word About Medications

Medications can lower your estrogen and testosterone levels by increasing your sex hormone-binding globulin (SHBG). This means that more of your natural hormones are bound to this carrier protein and aren't available to bind to the receptor to do you any good. The more of these hormones that are bound, the less activity they will have. Birth-control pills are one of the most significant medications for increasing SHBG. If you're fifty and taking the pill to prevent hot flashes, maybe it's time to stop, because there are better ways to do it. The most serious risks are heart attack, stroke, and blood clots. The risks increase if you smoke.

Progesterone

When hormones decline as we age, progesterone levels drop first and fastest. In contrast, estrogen falls only about 40 percent in the perimenopausal years. When you stop ovulating (in menopause), production of progesterone falls off a cliff. We want to ensure that we have adequate progesterone levels to balance estrogen's growth (proliferation) potential.

Progesterone-Friendly Foods

Increasing consumption of vitamin-B-rich foods boosts progesterone levels, as does decreasing saturated fats. If you eat meats and animal-product foods like dairy, you can wind up with a hormone imbalance, because animals are fed growth hormones today to fatten them up fast. Organic meat is from animals that haven't been given hormones, so choose organic and grass-fed beef whenever possible.

Wild yam is famous for containing hormone-like compounds that are very similar to progesterone, and it may encourage the body's own production of the hormone. You need to ensure that you do not choose sweet potato mistakenly. Sweet potatoes look like yams but do not have the same properties.

Herbs, Vitamins, and Other Options for Progesterone

Here are my recommendations for patients:

- ✧ **Chasteberry.** This herb raises progesterone levels.
- ✧ **Turmeric.** The spice, which is found in curry, helps increase progesterone levels. So do thyme and oregano.
- ✧ **Vitamin C** seems to improve progesterone. It's water-soluble, so it's safe to take, and you don't have to worry

about having too much. Your body gets rid of the excess through your urine.

◇ **Selenium** contributes to the production of progesterone.

Lifestyle

Stress is another factor in imbalance. Stress produces the hormone cortisol, which blocks the progesterone you do have from its receptor, preventing progesterone from getting where it needs to go in order to do its work. Overeating lowers progesterone levels, too. Progesterone is also produced in the adrenals and is really hard to make when the adrenals are busy combating stress. Progesterone is synthesized from pregnenolone, which is derived from cholesterol. Cholesterol is the reservoir for making all of our steroid hormones, including testosterone. Low cholesterol is a problem, although it's never been talked about that way. In fact, people brag about it. Yet suicide and homicide are higher in people who have very low cholesterol. High cholesterol isn't what we thought it was. It seems to be a message about inflammation in the body, and the fact that high cholesterol isn't the end of the story. What actually matters is the size of the molecules and how sticky they are. These factors are more important than our cholesterol number.

The Thyroid Connection

Balancing your thyroid hormones has a place in this discussion, because the thyroid gland is the conductor of the entire hormonal orchestra. Your hormones, and your body in general, aren't going to function at their best unless you have a thyroid that works well. There are many different thyroid hormones, such as T1, T2, T3, and T4, and the thyroid plays a big role in weight loss. People have the crazy idea that if they take thyroid medication they'll lose weight. It is not that simple. If you don't have an optimally functioning thyroid, your weight-loss efforts are unlikely to be successful. A thyroid in prime condition ensures that the pounds will drop off. I will discuss your thyroid in depth in the next chapter on adrenal glands, which affect the performance of thyroid hormones.

PART TWO

Building the Foundation for a Better Body, Brain, and Life

CHAPTER 4

Heal Your Adrenal Glands

L et me introduce you to your adrenal glands, two tiny glands the size of walnuts that sit on top of the kidneys. The adrenals are best known for releasing the hormone cortisol, which is often called "the stress hormone." But in truth the adrenals do so much more. They produce testosterone, estrogen, progesterone, and DHEA—especially after childbearing age, when the ovaries have completed their job.

In the world of sports and athletics, it's well known that the adrenal hormones known as steroids affect muscular strength and endurance. The adrenals also affect skin, blood pressure, blood sugar, sleep, the immune system, and electrolyte balance. If you've noticed your waist expanding as you get older, you can blame the adrenals' impact on the distribution of fat. These glands even affect cardiovascular and gastrointestinal functioning. No wonder your entire state of health suffers when the adrenals perform poorly.

Why am I telling you all this? Because in the last ten years a condition called adrenal fatigue has become one of the most common and widely missed threats to our well-being. Yet adrenal fatigue is frequently misdiagnosed, or, worse, missed as a diagnosis, despite being present in medical literature since the 1800s.

Adrenal fatigue is a collection of symptoms that affect multiple body systems and can wreck your quality of life. Do you feel tired instead of refreshed when you wake in the morning and drag yourself around throughout the day? Do you experience the 3 p.m. crash? Are you grumpy or depressed? Are you gaining weight even though you are not eating more or exercising less? If you answered yes to one or more of these questions, you may be battling this condition. Adrenal fatigue drains your hormones, causing deficiencies that can turn your life upside down. Even a mild case prevents you from looking and feeling your best.

I'm going to show you how to heal your adrenals and help them manufacture more of the hormones that fill you with energy and vitality. With time and the necessary ingredients, you can restore your adrenals to health so that they can do the job nature intended.

Adrenal Fatigue and the Cortisol Effect

Stress is the No. 1 cause of adrenal fatigue. But I'm talking about how we deal with stress, rather than about stress itself. It isn't stress that kills us; it's our reaction to it. The hormone cortisol, which the body pumps at the first sign of stress, messes us up. Your adrenal glands also do not know *how* to differentiate between various kinds of stress. They can't distinguish a wedding from a funeral.

In prehistoric times, cortisol helped us respond to life-or-death threats. If a great big bear suddenly appeared, the adrenals responded by secreting cortisol, which supplied the adrenaline burst you needed to run for your life like a track star. The cortisol secretion was supposed to last for about two minutes. By that time, either you became the bear's tasty lunch or you escaped. But that was then. Today, we live in a society where stress assaults us all day long—on the way to work, on the job, at home, and every time we pick up the newspaper or turn on the TV news. Our adrenals pump cortisol into our bodies for hours on end—every day.

Unfortunately, the adrenal glands respond not only to actual stress but also to the perception of stress, which starts when you wake up in the morning. Think about it. You open your eyes at 6 or 7 or 8 a.m. and face a new day filled with challenges. For many women, that jolt is quickly followed by slapping the adrenal glands awake with caffeine on an empty stomach, and by driving in traffic (or taking a train commute) to work. When you arrive, the stress continues. You may be late (or not). You check your email and find 130 messages waiting for you. Which are urgent? Only one way to find out. Meetings, phone calls, people, and deadlines follow, and the stress goes on and on. You eat lunch, but it's unlikely that you eat wholesome foods, sitting in a quiet place, fully present in the eating process. You are probably on your phone or computer checking email or Facebook. The fluorescent lights you're under all day long also add stress. Nature meant for us to get outdoors for fresh air and sunlight.

If you're a stay-at-home mom (SAHM), your stress is no less present. Household management, child care, chauffeuring the kids to their activities, meals, maid service, and social organizing often fill the entire day. My patients who are SAHMs often eat worse than women who work outside the home, because they have no defined breaks in the day. I remember when I had my first daughter. I realized that I no longer even went to the bathroom alone.

In response to this barrage of stress, your adrenal glands are so busy pumping out cortisol they don't have time to produce other important hormones you need—mainly DHEA, and androstenedione (the precursor of testosterone) and estrogen and progesterone. Your body receives constant messages of emergencies, and responds as if traffic, deadlines, and emails were matters of life and death. The result of all the cortisol secretion is adrenal fatigue, which exacts a big price.

Excess cortisol has been shown in studies to suppress the immune system, increase blood sugar, and create inflammation. Inflammation is believed to be the source of all conditions and diseases that make us sick and kill us, including cancer. Excess cortisol also affects two important processes in our bodies: catabolic metabolism and anabolic metabolism. The catabolic process breaks down muscle and other tissue. The anabolic process repairs and rebuilds tissue. If you have large amounts of cortisol surging through your body non-stop, your breakdown processes will exceed your repair processes, resulting in weaker bones and muscles and increased inflammation.

The Myth of Watching TV to Relax

Many of us get home from work exhausted and ready to relax. We plop down on the sofa and watch TV or grab a laptop and go on Facebook. But that doesn't heal the stress of the day or help you recuperate from its effects. Stress is a constant insult to your cells, creating inflammation through the release of cortisol and certain chemicals. The shot of cortisol was not supposed to last all day. Although watching TV stops the stress and helps you transition from stress to the absence of stress, it doesn't heal the wound. It won't help you take the important next step to rejuvenation. In order to turn back the clock and heal from the stress of the day, you actually need to *do* something.

We live in a society that has depleted its hormones at a much earlier stage than happened in the past. We contend with a chaotic world of change and heavier workloads, where even our playing is not restorative. Relaxing requires more than sitting passively in front of a screen. You have to activate the relaxation response, which was defined in the 1960s by the Harvard cardiologist Herbert Benson, MD. The relaxation response slows the heart rate, lowers blood pressure, and reduces oxygen consumption and cortisol levels. It is also associated with the release of hormones involved in the anabolic repair process. I prescribe stress-reducing practices like belly-breathing exercises, meditation, tai chi, guided imagery, and qigong to my patients to turn on the healing chemicals associated with the relaxation response.

RHYTHM OF CORTISOL LEVELS AND FATIGUE

Normally, your cortisol levels start rising in the very early morning and peak around 9 a.m. They then gradually drop from 3 p.m. to 9 p.m. and rise at 4 a.m. to start waking you up.

At first your body says, "Yeah, we can do this," when you're stressed—and pumps a ton of cortisol. But too much pumping of cortisol (in the acute stage of adrenal fatigue) eventually exhausts the adrenals, causing cortisol levels to drop dramatically. That's when people have a really hard time getting up in the morning and start feeling drowsy between 3 p.m. and 4 p.m. in the afternoon. You can't keep your eyes open unless you use a drug called caffeine, or sugar, to keep going. That is adrenal exhaustion. You're supposed to have a small decrease in cortisol production in mid-afternoon, but you're not supposed to crash. Some patients tell me that unless they're busy doing something, they literally fall asleep. They experience adrenal fatigue, where they need stimuli to keep themselves alert and present.

When your body is forced to produce cortisol all the time, it starts to run out of the ingredients needed to make it. That is when "cortisol steal" takes place. The adrenals "kidnap" the raw ingredients of other hormones (such as testosterone, progesterone, and estrogen) and use the ingredients to make more cortisol instead. It's a response to the constant command "There's stress, there's stress. You gotta produce more cortisol."

Not everyone experiences adrenal fatigue in exactly the same way. Some people have flat levels of cortisol all day long, causing constant fatigue. In others, cortisol levels rise at night, when they're supposed to be dropping down to allow sleep. As a result, these people can't fall asleep or can't stay asleep—and are exhausted in the morning. They feel their best and are most energetic after 9 p.m. or 10 p.m. at night.

Breathe Through Your Belly

I was a professional ballet dancer before I attended medical school in my thirties. Dancers are never allowed to breathe from the belly, and a tight-fitting tutu doesn't help. I was told to breathe through my rib cage. Yet if you look at young children you'll see that they breathe through the belly naturally. The diaphragm contracts and actually allows the lungs to fill with air, because it pulls the lungs down and creates a negative pressure. The belly actually expands.

Belly-breathing exercises are a powerful way to relieve stress and turn on the relaxation response. But our society's fashion norms and tight clothing have changed this normal breathing pattern to one where breath occurs in the chest and the shoulders. We women learned pretty young that having a flat tummy was sexy and beautiful. If we have a tummy we wear clothing, such as elasticized underwear, that prevents proper breathing.

The goal of getting a four-pack or a six-pack at the gym is what I call a muscular girdle. It holds us in, preventing diaphragmatic breathing. There's an upside to having rock-hard stomach muscles as a strong core for your back and posture. But some women go to extremes. Body image affects breathing these days.

Belly breathing has so many advantages. It increases rest and recuperation, resistance to infection, and circulation to non-vital organs like the skin. (Yes, you can actually improve your skin just by breathing!) These exercises also relieve headaches, decrease heart rate and blood pressure, and can prevent or help manage diabetes, because the adrenal glands play an important part in balancing our sugars. Sugars jump in a stress response because you need a burst of sugar to run away from the bear.

Belly breathing works because the vagus nerve, which attaches to the bottom of the diaphragm, directs the parasympathetic (as opposed to the sympathetic "fight or flight") nervous system. This system's purpose is rejuvenation and digestion. Belly breathing cools down all the inflammation produced by nonstop cortisol secretion, and shields cells from stress. The cooldown ideally happens every single day to turn on healing. Otherwise, your adrenal glands, those poor little walnut-size glands dealing with the response that never rests, say, "Seriously?" and partially shut down. They're like little gerbils repeating, "I'm doing the best I can."

Eventually, even your cortisol secretion plummets, because the adrenals are all worn out. Cortisol deficiency leads to fatigue, poor stress tolerance, hypersensitivity to the environment (particularly noise), absentmindedness, confusion, depression, anxiety, irritability, trouble with concentration, and more.

Belly-Breathing Exercise
The best way to start belly breathing is to:

1. Lie on the floor, with knees bent or a pillow under your knees. Put one hand on your chest and the other palm down on or near your belly.

2. Inhale through your nose, ensuring that your belly rises at least as high, if not higher than, your chest. Your reaction may be "That's hard!" But it's easy for children. That's the way we are designed to breathe. Look at a baby and you'll see that the belly goes up and the belly goes down. The chest and shoulders do not move. This allows oxygenation to go everywhere.

3. Each inhale should last for a count of four. Hold for seven seconds, and exhale for eight seconds. If you can't exhale for a full eight seconds, at least make sure you exhale longer than you inhale. Eventually, you can graduate to doing these exercises in a chair after you have trained your body to breathe lower than your chest and shoulders (or if you are in a location where you cannot lie down). I call this "Take Five."

I issue this challenge to my patients: "Ideally, I want you to do breathing exercises twice a day for ten minutes." They look at me and roll their eyes, as if I had asked them to fly to the moon. I know that's not going to happen. So I say to them—and to you, "Okay, we're going to do Take Five, as I just described, five times a day: (1) Five breaths when you wake up (before you get out of bed). (2) Five breaths before breakfast. (3) Five before lunch. (4) Five before dinner. (5) And, again, before you go to bed. We need to have a whole different conversation if you don't have time to take five breaths before you eat and when you wake up and go to bed."

You can even take one to two breaths at every red light if driving is something you do routinely. Create mental reminders every time you stop at a light (or eat or hang up the phone). The opportunities for these reminders linked to everyday activities are endless.

Stress is part of our lives. There's no avoiding it. But even a minute or two of belly breathing is beneficial.

Meditation

The National Center for Complementary and Alternative Medicine (NCCAM) defines meditation as a mind-and-body practice. There are many forms, and some involve practicing mindfulness of thoughts, feelings, and sensations without judgment. Mental and physical strategies help reduce wandering thoughts and perceptions and allow you to be present in the moment. You must take time out from the rest of the world and refresh, which is why meditation steadies you and connects you to your core.

When I suggest meditation to my patients, many respond, "Oh, that's hard." But I'm talking about a very basic meditation. If you haven't meditated before, start with ten minutes on the couch "sitting silently in stillness." Focus on the here and now, and give yourself plenty of time to become accustomed to it. Move up to twenty minutes as you get better at it. You stick with everything that is worth doing in your life. Be patient and allow yourself to improve little by little. Many of the world's most successful people (both financially and spiritually) have a daily meditation practice. You can, too.

Patients often ask whether they need to meditate every day, and I tell them the story of my dentist. When I was in grade school, I asked him if I had to floss all my teeth. "Only the ones you want to keep," he replied. The answer is similar for you. You only have to meditate on days when you want to heal the stress of that day.

What's that got to do with cortisol, testosterone, and other hormones? A whole lot, according to a 1997 study in the journal *Psychoneuroendocrinology*. This research compared levels of cortisol, testosterone, growth hormone, and thyroid-stimulating hormone before and after four months of a Transcendental Meditation (TM) program for one group of subjects versus a stress-education program for a control group. Basal and average cortisol levels dropped in the TM group, but not in the control. This supports previous data suggesting that repeated TM reverses the effects of chronic stress. In addition, testosterone levels increased in the TM group, along with levels of growth hormone and thyroid hormone.

A 2013 study in the journal *Psychological Science* found that mindfulness training may actually help boost test scores and improve working memory, too. Researchers at the University of California, Santa Barbara assigned forty-eight college students to a two-week mindfulness class—or to a nutrition class that met four times a week for forty-five minutes. The mindfulness class taught strategies to maintain focus and required the students to practice mindfulness in their daily activities. Mindfulness students had higher memory capacity and higher accuracy on the GRE test—an average sixteen-percentile-point boost. They had less mind wandering than the nutrition students and improved reading comprehension and working memory capacity.

Meditation improves brain and heart health, helps intuition and sleep, increases neuropathways, the ability to learn, and memory. It's an antidote for anxiety, anger, depressed feelings, and so much more.

Guided imagery, which offers vocal instructions as you practice, is a form of meditation and is easier for people who have a hard time with meditation.

One of the latest randomized, controlled studies on meditation suggests that the practice can even prevent full-blown high blood pressure. The study, published in 2013 in the journal *Psychosomatic Medicine,* followed fifty-six men and women averaging fifty years old with prehypertensive blood-pressure levels. It found that the meditation group had a greater reduction of blood pressure than the control group, which received progressive muscle relaxation instead. Meditation may actually reduce the need for medication.

Instead of life being a series of things that happen to us, meditation allows us to make choices. If you talk to actors in martial-arts movies and ask them, "How did you do that so fast?" they'll say, "It's like I'm in slow motion." Their brains have been trained to slow down, and it's as if they experienced spaces between moments. In those spaces is freedom of choice. That is part of meditative practice. Even though you are taking time out from your busy day to meditate, you will feel as if you have more time afterward, because you'll appreciate the time more.

And meditative practice depends on repetition. Every day I hear from my patients, "I'm not good at that." And I think, "Of course. You've never done it before." Can you imagine a baby saying, "I'm no good at walking"? Of course you're not good at it. But we know from neuropsychology that the brain is plastic, which means it can be molded and shaped. It's kind of like a muscle. You can make it do whatever you want it to—with repetition over time.

If you can't make meditation work for you, you might want to try meditation for the busy via Holosync, an aural system of meditation from the Centerpointe Research Institute, which discovered tones that we can't really hear. The system, which is based on real science and was created in 1989, puts the brain into an alpha-theta brain-wave pattern that stimulates the brain in the same way veteran meditators do. But it accelerates the meditation process at the push of a button. If you're curious, you can look it up at here:

Let me share a recent conversation I had with Bill Harris, the director of the Centerpointe Institute. Bill has been meditating for sixteen years and was inspired to find a way to meditate that was realistic for our twenty-first-century lifestyle. Bill told me that Holosync meditation "creates tremendous awareness that shows up as very specific brain changes. The changes result in the ability to observe your own internal processes that create how we feel, behave, and the people and situations we attract (or what is attracted to us), the meanings we assign as they happen and their consequences."

Life is impermanent and full of changes. The problem is we become attached to things in our lives. Most people do this on autopilot, outside of their awareness. If we increase our awareness, we increase our choice. Holosync research shows that the system increases creativity, mental clarity, pattern recognition, and a sense of well-being. Cortisol levels decreased 40 percent, melatonin levels increased 97 percent, and DHEA rose.

We all have stress. Some people experience the same workday you do and take it in stride. They have perspective. They take the long view. They breathe through the stressful moments. We all look at them and say, "Look at you. How are you able to handle all this?" Some of them are just genetically predisposed to type B personalities. Some have to develop these skills.

Other activities can help as well. There is even a lazy man's yoga called Thai massage, where you're stretched while you're fully clothed. Qigong (pronounced "chi gong") is an ancient healing art that involves controlled breathing and movement exercises designed to improve physical and mental well-being. Tai chi is another enormously helpful option. You can take classes in these activities or buy tapes for use at home.

The Sleep Factor and Your Adrenals

The adrenals are difficult to heal, because they're also affected by factors other than stress, such as the sleep cycle—not only how much you sleep but when you go to bed. The case of my patient Amy, a forty-nine-year-old physician with two young children, is a good example. She came to see me complaining of feeling tired all the time. "I don't know what's wrong with me," she told me. Ordinarily that wouldn't seem unusual, considering that she had a busy practice and two children—ages two and four—at home. But she added, "I try to work out, but if I do more than a walk I'm even more exhausted the next day. I get dizzy when I stand up. I'm getting scared. I've always been able to push through." She was also gaining weight, despite a healthy diet most of the time, and seemed to crave salt, which, oddly, is one of the signs of adrenal fatigue. An imbalance of the adrenal hormone aldosterone is linked to salt craving.

I asked Amy to fill out the adrenal health questionnaire I give to patients (see page 91), which revealed moderate adrenal fatigue. We examined her lifestyle choices more closely, and her sleep pattern stood out in bold. Amy went to bed every night at 1 a.m., which didn't give her body enough time to stay at the stage of sleep that is needed for rest and rejuvenation. Her body's secretion of cortisol began to rise and wake her up around 4 a.m., lifting her closer and closer to the surface of consciousness. Because she went to sleep so late, she got only three good hours of sleep. No wonder she had no energy in the morning.

Amy took a salivary cortisol test, which showed that her cortisol

THE FIVE STAGES OF SLEEP

How much you sleep and when you sleep affect the adrenals and the rest and repair action of your body. We cycle among five stages of sleep. These stages are grouped into two sleep patterns: REM and non-REM. REM sleep is the stage of rapid eye movement and is when we dream. Non-REM is the stage when our brain emits delta waves (the brain waves in deep, dreamless sleep) and is the deep sleep in which our bodies perform their restorative functions.

Stage 1. Our sleep begins with a stage of relaxed wakefulness where the eyes relax and our bodies release stress. This usually lasts from five to ten minutes. We then enter a state of drowsiness. People awakened during this stage will often deny that they were sleeping.

Stage 2. This stage lasts about twenty minutes and is associated with muscles alternating between relaxing and tensing.

Stage 3. This is the first stage of deep, non-REM sleep, when delta wave patterns begin. The delta waves are different from the alpha-theta brain waves seen in meditation.

Stage 4. This is the full-on delta phase, when bedwetting and sleepwalking occur for some people. The body then alternates between Stages 3 and 4 before entering Stage 5.

Stage 5. This is REM sleep, the stage where you dream. Your voluntary muscles are actually paralyzed now. Stage 5 is the one that many people skip, and is negatively affected by prescription sleep medications.

---

levels were flat all day. Normally, they should be high in the morning—to help us wake and deal with the day—and drop in the afternoon.

There is disagreement in the medical literature about the effects of sleep stages. Some people say the REM stage is the one you need in order to feel rested when you wake up in the morning. Others say you won't feel restored unless you get enough Stage 4 time. What it adds up to is: You need all five stages of sleep for rest and rejuvenation, just as you need the whole symphony of hormones working together.

The first step was to change Amy's bedtime from 1 a.m. to 10:30 p.m. I prescribed Cortisol Manager (Integrative Therapeutics), an over-the-counter herbal adrenal-replacement supplement that acts to support the adrenal glands at night.

To help Amy recover from stress and turn on the relaxation response, I prescribed the Take Five belly-breathing exercises. Amy also started meditating, although she had a problem with the word "meditation," because it seemed at odds with her religious beliefs. After just three months of changing her bedtime, along with supplementation and meditation, she lost five pounds and was more rested and energetic. She was beginning to feel like herself again.

The Nutrition Connection

What and when you eat are factors in adrenal fatigue as well. I put my adrenal patients on a program that includes foods to avoid, foods to eat, protein in the morning, good fats (yes, you need to eat fat to be fit), and timed snacks. When your blood sugar dips from skipping breakfast or postponing lunch until late in the afternoon, your body experiences stress and cortisol levels rise to compensate. Your brain requires glucose, which is the only food it uses, and your body will do whatever it takes to provide it.

Acidic Versus Alkaline Foods

I want my adrenal patients to load up on alkaline foods, such as green vegetables and many fruits, and avoid acidic foods. Alkaline foods help heal your adrenals, keep them running smoothly, provide an instant energy boost, and lower inflammation. Unfortunately, we become acidic as we age.

In 1931, Otto Warburg won the Nobel Prize in Physiology for his findings that cancer cells thrive in an acidic environment but cannot survive in an alkaline environment. He reported that cancer cells maintain a lower pH level than normal cells (as low as 6.6), due to the production of lactic acid and CO_2 (carbon dioxide). The term "pH" is a measure of the acidity of a substance. A pH of less than 7 is considered acidic. A pH greater than 7 is alkaline.

A higher pH level indicates a higher concentration of oxygen molecules; lower pH means a lower concentration of oxygen. I'm a huge fan of green juices and smoothies, because they create an alkaline environment for your cells. Oxygen-rich nutrients and green vegetables counteract the adrenal glands' secretion of their pro-inflammatory cascade. When my patients start juicing and using green smoothies, they can't believe how much better and more energetic they feel.

When Amy came to see me for a later checkup, she reported, "I'm a little better, but not great." She was a perfectionist who expected to be successful 100 percent of the time.

I asked her to send me a food diary of everything that went into her mouth for three days. Like many women, Amy had an "all or nothing" attitude. If she succumbed to pizza for lunch, she'd throw away her regimen for the rest of the day. "You don't have to eat perfectly," I told her. "Life isn't an unwavering line but a meandering path."

We followed with an extensive nutritional consultation about alkaline foods and foods rich in vitamin C, which are beneficial for the adrenals. They include colored vegetables and fruit, sprouts (sunflower, alfalfa, and clover). In general, the younger the plant the more vitamin C it contains. Amy hadn't strictly followed these recommendations, either. She was cutting corners.

In a case like this, I also advise eating lightly cooked or raw protein when possible. This preserves amino acids and the naturally occurring enzymes needed to digest foods, thus decreasing the body's workload. My suggestions for protein included sashimi, seviche, steak tartare, legumes combined with whole grains, and seeds or nuts.

I also reminded Amy that the body's response to stress is to put on lots of belly fat. Many people find it a challenge to lose weight, especially around the waist.

After asking a few questions, I discovered that Amy was not meditating as agreed. People always tell me they don't have time to meditate. But that's like going to bed without brushing your teeth. Stress is the food in our teeth. We must brush and floss the stress out of our bodies to prevent damage to our cells.

Amy agreed to try differently (not harder) and left with new motivation. Recently, she told me that she feels better than she has since college. She's able to get through the day with optimism, although she isn't 100 percent and can get tired. She still has trouble giving up eating and sleeping patterns she used to get away with. But now she feels energized most days. I encouraged her to continue. For some people, it can actually take up to two years for the adrenals to fully heal. Amy probably had adrenal fatigue in medical school, and she's a mom with two kids. Her medical issues have been building for years.

Over-the-Counter Supplements for Adrenal Fatigue

If you have adrenal fatigue, you're going to have to supplement your diet with specific vitamins and minerals, especially vitamin C, to aid in healing your adrenals. You can't get enough vitamin C by eating oranges, and I don't recommend orange juice or fruit juices; they are liquid candy. These are hard on the adrenals, because they cause a sugar blast, and then you crash.

Here are the over-the-counter products I recommend to my patients:

DO YOU HAVE ADRENAL FATIGUE?

Below is a list of common symptoms of adrenal fatigue. To evaluate your own adrenal function, fill in the numbers at right that apply to you:

	AGREE (2)	AGREE SOMEWHAT (1)	DISAGREE (0)
1. I am constantly tired.	____	____	____
2. I have allergies.	____	____	____
3. I have asthma.	____	____	____
4. I get sick often.	____	____	____
5. I am under severe emotional stress.	____	____	____
6. I suffer from chronic pain or other physical stress.	____	____	____
7. I have low blood pressure.	____	____	____
8. I have a hard time getting out of bed every morning.	____	____	____
9. When I rise quickly, I get light-headed momentarily.	____	____	____
10. I crave salt or salty foods.	____	____	____
11. I would feel better if I could sleep until 9 a.m.	____	____	____

Total Score: ____

If your score is over 8 it is likely you have adrenal fatigue.

Vitamins

✧ **Vitamin B Supplements**
a) **Vitamin B3.** This has been shown to support the adrenal glands.
b) **Vitamin B6.** It's been said that if you have trouble recalling your dreams you might have a B6 deficiency.
c) **Vitamin B12.** Supports adrenal function.
d) **Niacin.** Has been shown to support adrenal function. Niacin has a tendency to make you feel flushed (turn red and tingle). You can buy the "non-flushing" type (it says that on the label), or many people take a baby aspirin before the niacin to diminish the flushing.
e) **Pantothenic Acid.** This is for energy production and is present in all cells. However, much higher quantities are found in the adrenals, because so much energy is needed to produce adrenal hormones. Pantothenic acid with magnesium, vitamin E, and vitamin C increases energy and takes much of the fatigue out of the adrenals without overstimulating them.
f) **Vitamin B Complex.** This has multiple B vitamins in one pill.
✧ **Vitamin C.** This is probably the most important vitamin. The more cortisol secreted, the more vitamin C you need. It's water-soluble, which means you don't store it. Your body will excrete it in your urine if you take more than you need. It appears that vitamin C complex (rather than ascorbic acid) is most beneficial for the adrenals. Many people assume that ascorbic acid is vitamin C, but it's not. It's a portion of the vitamin C complex, and we don't know whether it's fully metabolized, recognized, and utilized by the body.

Be aware that ascorbic acid, which is often made from corn syrup, cane sugar, or beet sugar, is frequently sold over the counter as vitamin C. But corn syrup and sugar do not contain vitamin C.

These are just the raw ingredients of commercially manufactured vitamin C. If you have a sensitivity to corn, you might have a sensitivity to this commercially manufactured ascorbic acid. What you need are the bioflavonoids that are in vitamin C. If you're on blood thinners, high doses of vitamin C can change your blood clotting and coagulation, so you do have to be very careful. Keep this in mind if you're having surgery, including dental surgery, and stop taking vitamin C one week before the procedure.

✧ **Vitamin E.** This vitamin, as a mixed tocopherol (as found in nature), is an indirect requirement because it's needed in at least six different enzymatic reactions in the adrenal cascade. Adequate vitamin E (tocopherol is its technical name) is essential for the reaction to work properly.

Vitamin E serves another purpose, too. Manufacturing hormones in the adrenals actually generates a lot of free radicals, which are associated with cancer and can damage cells. Vitamin E neutralizes the free radicals inside the adrenal glands and elsewhere. Note that vitamin C enhances vitamin E's activity, and the two work hand in hand.

Most vitamin E sold in stores is in the form d-alpha tocopherol, which is only a portion of the complete vitamin E complex—and our body seems to know the difference. Manufacturers do this because it's the least expensive way to make vitamin E, and the most profitable. But studies show that these do not provide the same health benefits as mixed tocopherol. We really need mixed-tocopherol supplementation, one high in beta-tocopherol. Look at the label on the bottle. Caution: Vitamin E can affect blood clotting.

Minerals

✧ **Calcium Citrate or Calcium Lactate.** Calcium feeds the adrenals and calms the sympathetic nervous system (the fight-or-flight response).

- **Magnesium Citrate.** This is a spark plug for the adrenals, and is best taken before bed. Magnesium is also great for pain, muscle cramps, and headaches, which so many women experience. Epsom salts contain magnesium. Take a little tub with warm water, add Epsom salts, and soak your feet in it while watching TV. Your skin will absorb that magnesium and relieve any pain. Even better, add essential oil of lavender. Lavender has been shown to decrease anxiety and depression and to relieve the effects of stress.
- **Sodium.** Adrenal fatigue reduces the amount of aldosterone, the hormone that controls sodium and potassium in the body (and is secreted by the adrenals). Sodium balance can't be properly maintained. As a consequence, dehydration occurs even if you drink enough water. People with adrenal fatigue often crave salt. The best sources of salt are sea salt, kelp, green and black olives, red peppers, Swiss chard, beet greens, celery, and zucchini.
- **Trace Minerals.** You also need manganese, selenium, molybdenum, chromium, copper, and iodine. You can buy a mineral supplement that combines all of them. It has a calming effect on the body and is especially valuable if you're nervous or jittery.

Herbs

- **Ashwagandha.** If your cortisol level is too high, ashwagandha calms it down. If the cortisol level is too low, it boosts it. I prescribed ashwagandha for Amy.
- **Ginger.** Fresh ginger is anti-inflammatory and strengthens the adrenals. It also increases the metabolic rate and fat-burning. You can take it in tea.
- **Herbal Adrenal Cell Extracts.** Extracts are the oldest and most reliable way of healing the adrenals. They have been commercially available since the flu epidemic in the United States in 1918. Respiratory infections are especially hard on the adrenal

glands, and in 1919 Lucke and associates at Camp Zachary Taylor found that adrenal exhaustion was present in 103 of 126 autopsies performed on flu victims. The adrenals weren't infected, but they had to work so much harder. I prescribed this extract for Amy.

✧ **Licorice Root.** This herb gives black licorice its flavor and is great for the adrenal glands. It contains plant hormones that mimic the effect of cortisol, thus giving the adrenals a break from producing cortisol. Some adrenal patients crave licorice or salt. No, you don't have to eat candy. You can get licorice root in supplement form.

✧ **Siberian Ginseng Root.** This helps calm anxiety, increases energy, reduces irritability, and helps improve and increase your overall sense of well-being and your ability to handle stress. Look for ginseng with at least 0.8 percent of eleutherosides (the active ingredient). Caution: Siberian ginseng can have a stimulatory effect and is not recommended for people with high blood pressure.

Also:

✧ **DHEA.** This hormone is huge in adrenal-fatigue treatment, and is also available over the counter. DHEA is the raw ingredient of your hormones and an excellent indicator of your adrenal health. Studies show that a high DHEA level directly correlates with longevity. The adrenals manufacture 80 percent of DHEA and use DHEA to produce testosterone and other hormones.

✧ **Fiber.** When you experience adrenal fatigue, mild constipation is often present. Fiber, such as cellulose or pectin, will help. Just avoid any that contain lots of sugar and corn syrup. Be aware, too, that "sugar-free" isn't necessarily better for you. The chemical substitutes are even worse. Or have a green smoothie (with or without chia seeds) for your fiber.

Lifestyle Prescription

The foods, supplements, and exercises discussed in this chapter will help heal your adrenals. But lifestyle changes are also necessary to complete the job. This is what I want you to incorporate into your days and weeks ahead:

Laughter

A hearty laugh actually changes your brain waves and the chemistry of your body, and it does heal. I tell my patients to rent funny movies, and to laugh even if it seems insincere at first. Try it, and you'll see that it can start to become second nature.

Once a week minimum, spend time with friends. Make sure they're not "energy suckers," however. We all have people we care about a lot, but when we leave them we feel tired. They drain us. In order to be healthy and strong, you have to have boundaries. Get together with friends who make you feel energized after you see them—to heal your adrenals. Before you say yes to a social engagement, ask yourself, "Will this event and the people involved stress me or bless me?"

Recognize other energy robbers (like the phone) and eliminate those, too. Don't keep the cell on all the time. It seems we have a compulsion to check our phones, but we have to discipline ourselves to stop the phone from taking over our lives. The minute you keep checking your emails, you have surrendered your day to someone else's agenda, not yours. People say, "Oh, it's important, because someone may want to reach me." Yeah, it's important—for them, not for what you want to get done that day. If you set the intention, you do it. Check your email twice a day—that's all. Look at your phone twice a day. Never let electronic devices interrupt a conversation with a real human being.

Gratitude

We used to think love was the most powerful emotion. It isn't; it's gratitude. Find out what you're grateful for by paying attention.

Write down one thing you're grateful for every day. Send the words in an email to someone or write it down in a journal. Science makes it pretty clear that gratitude really changes your brain. We're finding out through positive psychology that happiness is a choice—and you can train your brain to be happy. Research shows that gratitude is one of the significant tools for boosting your own contentment. In one study, couples who told their partners three things they were grateful for about each other were seen to be more attractive after six months of doing this gratitude exercise. Who doesn't want to get better-looking?

The movie producer and serial entrepreneur Jeff Hays has created a wonderful way to make gratitude fun, with an app called Gratitapp. Jeff told me the story of how this app came to be. He was sitting writing in his daily gratitude journal all the things and people that he was grateful for that day. When he was done, he closed his book and looked out the window. He realized that all the people he had felt love and appreciation for in his journal for the day had no idea how he felt about them. The gratitude stopped when he closed the book. He wondered how it would affect people's lives to know how grateful he was for them. Enter the Gratitapp. When you write your gratitudes, the app automatically sends a gratitude message to those you included. Talk about spreading positive energy!

Movement

Don't forget to move. Park your car farther away from your destination so that you have to walk. Take the stairs instead of the elevator. These are little things that really add up. My neighbor is a busy surgeon in Seattle and has a lot going on. He's forty-three, and he's on medication for high cholesterol. While discussing the importance of movement and exercise, he said to me, "I thought of running, but I have no time." He gets up at 5 a.m. to make his rounds and dictate, followed by surgery. What he does do is turn on the shower in the morning. While it's warming up, he does push-ups and pull-ups and stretches. He says, "I know it's just four or five minutes, but it's really made a difference. I'm stronger."

I stretch my calves and hamstrings while I brush my teeth every day. It's built-in. I never forget, because brushing is my cue.

Thyroid and the Adrenal-Fatigue Connection

The same stress that causes adrenal fatigue can also create an underactive thyroid (hypothyroidism). People don't realize that adrenal fatigue and hypothyroidism are often linked. We already know that cortisol pours out when we have adrenal fatigue—and that cortisol is catabolic. It puts the body into a metabolic state of breaking down. When the thyroid, which is in charge of metabolism, sees the increase in catabolic metabolism, it slows down! Thyroid disease is the most poorly treated condition in conventional medicine, because often the symptoms of low thyroid are just like the symptoms of adrenal fatigue. The two are often confused. The problem is that if your doctor prescribes thyroid medication (and you have adrenal fatigue), you will feel no improvement—or feel worse. Feeling wired and tired is common when the thyroid but not the adrenal glands is treated. Another reason hypothyroidism is poorly treated is that the so-called "normal" range is as big as a house. In your twenties, you may have been at the top of the normal range. But now that you're in your forties you might drop to the bottom of your range. That dive can make an enormous difference in how you feel, although your doctor still considers you "normal."

We need to look at the thyroid from an optimal-functioning perspective. Women have an epidemic of thyroid problems today, and it could be caused by a lack of iodine. Iodine is essential to proper thyroid function, and we don't have enough in our diets. Iodine has also been shown to be protective against breast cancer. Iodine receptors are more abundant in breast tissue than elsewhere. Countries like Japan, where women work hard, smoke, drink, and are stressed, have

THYROID SELF-TEST

Do You Have Low Thyroid Function (Hypothyroidism)?

Below are the symptoms commonly found in thyroid deficiency. In each case below, fill in the number at right that applies to your situation:

	AGREE (2)	AGREE SOMEWHAT (1)	DISAGREE (0)
1. I'm sensitive to the cold, particularly in my hands and feet.	____	____	____
2. My face and eyelids are puffy in the morning.	____	____	____
3. I put on weight easily.	____	____	____
4. I have dry skin.	____	____	____
5. I have trouble getting up in the morning.	____	____	____
6. I feel more tired resting than when active.	____	____	____
7. I am constipated.	____	____	____
8. My joints are stiff in the morning.	____	____	____
9. I feel like I'm living in slow motion.	____	____	____
10. My palms and the soles of my feet are yellowish.	____	____	____

Total Score: ____

If your score is 6 or above, you have low thyroid.

a diet very high in iodine—and among the lowest risks of breast cancer. At anti-aging conferences, one of the things you hear is that you should take a low dose of iodine every day or take seaweed, because they are very protective against breast cancer.

Iodine was originally added to salt because we had a nationwide deficiency. However, culinary trends have led people to use sea salt, kosher, or other salts that do not contain iodine. It can be hard to find even ordinary table salt with iodine on supermarket shelves. People associate salt with being unhealthy. If they have high blood pressure or heart problems or are diabetic, they try to avoid salt. The thinking is that this great idea has caused unintended side effects in the form of thyroid problems.

Try to find a physician who knows how to treat thyroid and can get you into the optimal ranges safely and effectively.

Pamper Your Adrenals

Even if you don't have adrenal fatigue, you still want to keep your adrenals healthy and functioning well. Subpar adrenal glands undermine your body's hormone production as well as your general health. Your brain doesn't have a prayer if the hormones produced by the adrenals are too low to do their job. Balancing and increasing your hormones is actually a treatment for adrenal fatigue.

CHAPTER 5

Detoxify Your Liver

Chinese medicine has a saying: "Happy liver, happy life." And Hippocrates, the father of medicine, told us that good health begins in the liver and the digestive tract. Modern research has shown both statements to be true. Simply be nice to your liver and it will take good care of you. This superorgan acts as a processor for testosterone, estrogen, progesterone, and certain other hormones—plus any hormones your doctor may have prescribed. The liver activates these hormones, allowing them to start doing their work, and removes excess hormones that might cause an imbalance. Surplus hormones are as problematic as hormone deficiency.

The liver also filters out toxins and chemicals you ingest, absorb, and breathe every day—substances that interfere with hormones doing their job. Not many people associate the liver with hormones. Yet your hormone levels dive if filtering is sluggish. The liver breaks down hormones into a form that allows toxins to be excreted from the body. If the process doesn't work efficiently, the result can be hormone imbalance.

The mighty liver performs an anti-cancer function, too. Hormones can have cancer-causing properties, and an optimally functioning liver chemically changes many hormones to keep our cells safe.

In order to handle all these important tasks, the liver must be in top form. Yet risks to the liver are everywhere. This organ is forced to work overtime today, filtering the pollutants in the environment and the chemicals in our foods and in products ranging from hair conditioners to furniture. Lifestyle issues, and the anger and other emotions we must handle in our 24/7 society, also interfere with liver function. These stresses keep your liver scrambling, and often it is much too busy to process your hormones properly.

Although many people suffer from adrenal fatigue, absolutely everyone (including you and me) has a liver under siege. That's why there is no self-test in this book for the liver. We all need a restorative tune-up to keep our liver humming, and I urge my patients to do a metabolic liver cleanse at least once a year. Otherwise, all the toxins that a limping liver can't eliminate remain in the body and wind up traveling to the lungs, skin, kidneys, lymphatic system, and colon to do damage.

When the oil filter in your car stops working, you replace it with a new one. That's all it takes to fix the problem. But you can't do that with your poor liver. Instead, you need to detoxify, heal, cleanse, and rejuvenate the liver you've got. That's where the liver cleanse stands out.

Understanding the Detox System

Hormones manufactured by the adrenal glands, such as testosterone, estrogen, progesterone, plus thyroid and certain other hormones, go directly to the liver. There the hormones are processed in a two-part system. Let's see how it works.

Many of the toxins we're exposed to are fat-soluble, making their disposal from the body difficult or impossible. Phase 1 of the liver's detoxification (which is known as oxidation and uses the cyto-chrome P450 system) takes our hormones apart. Phase 1 takes lipid-soluble compounds, which are hard to excrete from the body, and makes the toxins more water-soluble for Phase 2.

The liver breaks down the hormones known as steroid hormones, which include:

✧ The sex hormones estrogen, progesterone, and testosterone, which control our body, shape, energy, and sex life.
✧ Aldosterone, which controls the balance of the minerals sodium and potassium as well as water in the body.
✧ Cortisone, which plays a significant role in the immune system (among many other functions).

That is only part of the detox story, however. Phase 1 also has a dark side. It can take a toxic substance and make it even more dangerous. The problem is that the metabolites, which are the end result

SIGNS OF LIVER PROBLEMS

There is a blood test for the liver called LFT. Unfortunately, the liver must be very sick for measurable signs of trouble to show up in this test. I don't want you to wait that long. Just be aware of these common symptoms of a sluggish liver:

❖ Unexplained weight gain
❖ Poor immune function
❖ High blood pressure
❖ Skin problems (remember your grandmother's liver spots?)
❖ High cholesterol
❖ Digestive problems
❖ Fatigue

Thankfully, the liver is a unique organ that is able to repair and regenerate new and healthy liver cells when it receives the right help.

of Phase 1, can sometimes be (a) very active, and (b) even more toxic than the original substance. That's why it's so important that Phase 2 detoxification, which is known as conjugation, occurs.

Phase 2 of the detox system reconfigures our hormones, adding molecules to the toxins left over from Phase 1. This process protects us from developing cancer and from the damages of inflammation. Unfortunately, Phase 2 of our detoxification system becomes less effective as we age. But you don't have to resign yourself to a sluggish liver. My comprehensive metabolic liver cleanse helps you power up detoxification for optimal health.

What Is the Liver Cleanse?

My liver cleanse takes two weeks, and I describe it as "sending your liver to the gym for fifteen days." It's a system of supplements, rich protein shakes, nourishing juices, specific menu choices (but not a diet), detoxification teas, and even bath soaks and skin scrubs. The cleanse consists of two parts, working simultaneously.

The first part, the elimination part, is felt mostly during the first three days (but continues throughout the cleanse). This part helps eliminate toxins from the liver through diet and certain over-the-counter supplements. Liver damage is not due only to pesticides on your lawn and fire retardants on the new mattress you bought. Supermarkets are filled with processed foods containing ingredients that sound as if they belong in a chemistry lab. I tell my patients, "If you can't pronounce the name of the ingredient you're eating, your liver probably can't figure it out, either."

The toxins drawn out by the cleanse are released into the bloodstream, temporarily causing many people (but not all) to feel tired, or as if they have the flu. The more toxins there are in your liver, the worse you're going to feel. Expect it, and just keep thinking about your liver gradually being restored to prime health. The liver is such an amazing organ that you can hack off half of it and it will grow back. But it needs your help now to stay strong.

Detox Through Elimination, Perspiration, and Body Scrubs

Remember, the point of Phase 1 detox is to create water-soluble toxins that are more easily removed by the body—and rejuvenate the liver itself. I give my patients a detoxification tea that encourages urination, in addition to helping with the breaking-down process. The more tea you drink, and the more you urinate, the more toxins you remove. An infrared sauna also plays a large role in detox, because toxins are removed by sweat as well as by urination. This type of sauna, available at many spas and gyms, enhances your circulation and helps oxygenate tissues. Your skin is a major organ of elimination, yet most of us don't sweat on a regular basis.

A type of infrared sauna called a far-infrared (FIR) sauna removes toxins safely and naturally. This sauna was also shown to lower both systolic (the top number) and diastolic (the bottom number) blood pressure in a 2005 randomized double-blind placebo-controlled study at the University of Missouri–Kansas City.

Because the skin also absorbs toxins and chemicals, I tell my patients to do a dry body scrub using a scrubbing mitt and Himalayan salt, which is available at many health-food stores or at your local spa. A scrub before showering or bathing stimulates the lymphatic system, circulation, and helps exfoliation. It not only aids the detox process but also leaves your skin glowing!

The last place toxins exit the body is through your breath, which may not be your best feature for a week or so. You're going to have bad breath. It's part of the process, although you can eat cloves or mint leaves if you like. You can also chew gum or use mints sweetened with stevia.

Nutrition and the Cleanse

Remember that I spoke of the liver cleanse as a two-part process. The second part focuses on nutritional changes designed to heal individual cells in the liver, called the kupffer cells, and improve their function. During the cleanse, you choose from an approved list of liver-friendly foods. Foods to eat include a wide variety of fruits and vegetables, most nuts, most fish, chicken, turkey, lamb, rice, potatoes, certain grains like quinoa, olive oil, and more.

Banned foods include grapefruit, corn, foods containing gluten, soybeans and soy products, peanuts, tuna and swordfish and shellfish, milk, butter, cheese, eggs, yogurt, caffeinated coffee, chocolate, sugar, mayonnaise, and more. Tomatoes and some other nutritious foods are excluded because they're processed through the liver—and the cleanse is designed to reduce work for this exhausted organ and give it a break. Alcohol is out for the same reason. See the complete list of approved and banned foods on pages 150–151 in Chapter 7. Alkaline foods, which include green vegetables and many fruits, heal not only the adrenal glands but your liver, too.

A metabolic liver cleanse actually saved one of my patients from undergoing a liver biopsy last year. Janine, a forty-six-year-old divorced dentist, had gone to her primary-care physician for a checkup, presenting no complaints other than fatigue. After testing, the doctor found that her liver enzymes were slightly elevated. He asked about her drinking and drug history. Janine didn't use drugs or abuse alcohol, although she enjoyed three or four drinks a week. She exercised and had above-average, healthy eating habits. "Well, we'll just watch it," the doctor told her.

Janine left her doctor's office with the instructions to "wait and see"—and no real plan. She subsequently came to see me to try a different approach to get her energy back. I gave her a blood test, which showed that she had an elevated level of ferritin (stored iron) in her liver. Her liver enzymes had risen from slightly elevated to

WATCH OUT

Other substances affect the ratio of Phase 1 to Phase 2 and impede the delicate balance between the two. Those that hurt your Phase 1 detox system include:

❖ Alcohol
❖ Charbroiled meat
❖ Saturated fats
❖ Grapefruit*
❖ Nicotine
❖ Medications such as antihistamines and steroids
❖ Pesticides

Conditions that hurt your Phase 2 detox system include:

❖ Deficiencies in vitamin C, B1, B5, and B12, and in selenium, zinc, magnesium, choline, and folic acid.

Your regular doctor doesn't check the activity of your liver-detox system, so you should assume that you don't have a perfect liver. That's why it's so important to do the liver cleanse.

---

*Grapefruit slows down the metabolism of some drugs through the liver by up to 30 percent. That's why your doctor tells you not to eat grapefruit when taking certain medications.

moderately elevated. I did more tests, and sent the results to her primary-care physician, who now wanted Janine to get a liver biopsy. Distraught at the thought of having somebody stick a needle in her liver, Janine returned to see me. "This isn't just a flu shot," she said. "I'm terrified."

I totally sympathized, and suggested postponing the biopsy and trying a liver cleanse first. "Let's see what happens after the cleanse," I told her. However, this cleanse would take three weeks (rather than the fifteen-day regimen followed by my other patients) because Janine's liver was in worse shape than the usual liver. "We'll reevaluate after the cleanse," I assured her. "If the cleanse works as I hope, you may not need the biopsy. But the cleanse won't have a chance unless you strictly follow the regimen. No cheating. You need to suck it up," I told her bluntly.

The cleanse is not overly restrictive, and Janine agreed to make the commitment. She stuck to the regimen.

In addition to the recommended foods, Janine drank four glasses of organic green juices a day to bathe her kupffer cells in nutrients. She took the easy route and made a big batch in the morning, divided it up, and poured it into Mason jars. Late in the afternoon, she made another big batch and saved it for the evening. I'm a big fan of organic juicing and smoothies. For example, cucumbers, celery, kale, carrots, apples, and organic coconut water can be churned up to the consistency you want for a liver-friendly midmorning snack.

Herbs and Supplements

Liver-friendly nutrition is critical to the detox process, but it can't do the job alone. Over-the-counter supplementation is also necessary for the detox process, and to help heal liver cells.

Herbs that heal and detoxify the liver include:

⬧ **Fenugreek.** Research has found it to be a protective agent for the liver.
⬧ **Marshmallow Root.** This is most commonly used for respiratory issues and can decrease inflammation in the liver.
⬧ **Milk Thistle.** This herb has been used for two thousand years for a range of liver problems. It protects the liver cells by reinforcing

the cell membranes, renewing liver cells, and clearing free radicals from the liver. It may also lower LDL (bad) cholesterol.

✧ **Slippery Elm.** This aids in the elimination process through the gastrointestinal (GI) tract.

✧ **Turmeric.** This is used to treat liver problems and is anti-inflammatory.

Several studies show that the liver-friendly supplement phosphatidylcholine can also help your memory and brain. As women get older, they say, "I'm not as sharp as I used to be." Phosphatidylcholine, which is often erroneously confused with lecithin, is called the power brain-boosting supplement.

In Janine's case, I prescribed my proprietary detox protein. Nothing can keep toxins away from the liver, but this and the protein called MediClear are very good at drawing them out.

When I retested Janine seven days after she'd completed the cleanse, the results were startling. Her liver enzymes and everything else fell within normal range. Although she lost only a few pounds, she said she felt lighter. That's pretty typical in people who do the cleanse. It's as if the toxins weighed you down internally. Most important, there was no longer any reason for Janine to have a liver biopsy. In the past five years, many of my patients have had the same experience. In the earliest days of medicine, food was used to heal. This works today as well. If you give your liver what it needs to heal and detox, it will!

As for the iron stored in Janine's liver, it turned out that she had cooked daily in a cast-iron pot. The metal she absorbed had caused her to accumulate iron, mimicking a genetic disorder of the liver called hemochromatosis. Symptoms include chronic fatigue and joint pain. I told her to stop using cast-iron cookware immediately, and put her on a low-iron diet that excludes foods like red meat, spinach, raisins, and beans. I continue to monitor her.

THE ALCOHOL AND
MEDICATION FACTORS

Alcohol is not only toxic to a struggling liver; it's lethal. When your liver detoxifies wine, beer, and liquor, it puts other tasks on hold (even when you have one glass of Chardonnay). Why? Everything else must wait, because just one glass of wine can kill you if it isn't detoxified by the liver.

Research has also found that your liver can "up-regulate." If you have one or two glasses of wine every single night, your liver says, "Okay. I'm good." It's gone to the "alcohol gym" and can handle alcohol if you drink on a regular basis. But when you move up to three or more glasses, your liver says, "You must be kidding." Three or more seems to be the tipping range.

But the very worst thing you can do is abstain during the week and gulp six drinks a night on the weekend. Your liver can't handle binge drinking. It's too much in one isolated dose.

I want everyone to know, however, that alcohol is not healthy. A lot

The Emotional Tie-In

Certain emotions, such as anger and resentment, can be toxic to your liver as well. In fact, Chinese medicine calls the liver "the seat of anger." These feelings must be put into perspective if your liver is to do its job right. Research shows that situations or relationships that make you feel powerless create the most stress. You can be in a difficult spot, but as long as you feel you have some ability to change it, you don't feel stressed out.

Do you react with frustration and anger if someone else takes credit for your work or you miss out on a raise or the car breaks down? Or do you respond with a deep breath and a sense of perspec-

of attention has been paid to the ingredient in red wine called resveratrol, which is good for the heart. The truth is that the amount of wine you'd need to consume in order to get a therapeutic dose of resveratrol is way too much to be healthy. I consider wine to be a tolerable indulgence, like sugar. Don't fool yourself into thinking that alcohol is healthy. It is not. But a small amount once in a while is unlikely to hurt you.

The Trouble with Medications

Prescription drugs can be another huge load on the liver. Many meds slow down Phase 1 of the detox system. For example, the antibiotic Cipro inhibits cytochrome P450, the enzyme responsible for detoxification. Try to picture this enzyme as the catcher in a baseball game. He is going to have a hard time performing if Cipro holds one of his arms behind his back and says, "Okay. Now try and do it. Catch the ball." The drugs Nexium, Prilosec, and a blood-pressure medication called verapamil have the same effect. So does grapefruit juice. I don't advocate that people stop taking their prescription medications. But when you're on them your liver needs more help—a cleanse.

tive? Those are choices. However, often we erupt before our brain can kick in. Having a hormone imbalance only makes matters worse. Many of my patients tell me they feel as if they are watching themselves react and their "choice" has been taken away. They ask me, "How can I slow things down?"

My reply is that the first step is noticing the tiniest ripple of rising anger—and taking a breath. Maybe instead of exploding you can remove yourself and say, "I'll be right back." You take a break and take a walk. Head for the bathroom and do the belly-breathing exercise that I described on page 81 in Chapter 4. Inhale for a count of four; hold for seven (whatever you can manage, because it can be hard to hold your breath); exhale for eight. Do it five times, and when you return the situation will look very different.

Often the initial response occurs because we personalize the situation and feel we're being singled out or that we're responsible. The reality is people don't have time to focus on us. They're trying to make their own life work and usually you just happen to be there. Yes, there are times when people are targeted, but that's the exception, not the norm. I know how difficult it can be to stay calm in times of stress and frustration.

It takes practice to keep your cool. The more you do it, the better you become. And it circles back. If you do your breathing exercise and meditation, you also train your brain to react differently.

Timing for a Liver Cleanse

A liver cleanse is challenging, because it restricts your choices. The obvious limitation is in what you eat. But your social outings may be affected, too, if you feel uncomfortable about being the only one abstaining from a glass of wine or eating differently. Travel options might be affected. You need to take control of your food and buy or make medicinal juice, as well as make sure your day will allow you to take all your supplements and the cleansing protein shake. If you're hiking all day, that may not be the best time for a cleanse.

Business trips are probably the worst time, because your schedule is not your own. If you drink lots of detox tea, you're going to keep peeing. Will it be convenient to get up during a meeting or a conference session that's expected to last two or three hours? Probably not. And the whole point is to eliminate. You don't want to hold it.

Both Ayurvedic and Chinese medicine say that spring is the time to do a cleanse. I've found that the people I see are more interested in a cleanse in January, after the temptations of the holiday season are gone. January seems a good time to start fresh and heal the damage done by all those extra cocktails and the acidic and fatty foods you ate from Thanksgiving through New Year's Day.

However, I've recently started doing something different—a pre-cleanse in October to mid-November instead of after the holidays. I find that the body can handle the insult of Thanksgiving through New Year's because it starts at a better place. People make wiser choices during the holidays, because they look and feel better and don't want to ruin it. If you've lost three to five pounds, you hate to gain it back.

The pre-cleanse has worked extremely well for my patients. The best time for a cleanse is when you're going to be successful, which is when you can have control over your food. April tax season would be a horrible time for an accountant, because you can't have coffee during a liver cleanse.

How difficult is the cleanse? I just got an email from a patient who said, "My partner and I are on day ten of the liver cleanse, and, to be honest, it's not what we expected. We thought we'd feel a lot lousier, and have to spend all day in the bathroom. It was much easier than that." She had confused a liver cleanse with a colon cleanse, which really is awful. It's like preparing for a colonoscopy. A liver cleanse isn't in the same category.

In fact, I don't think the colon needs to be cleansed. The colon is our pipeline and plumbing. Lots of good bacteria need to live in there. If you completely cleanse it out with colon therapy and coffee enemas, you hurt the environment of those good bacteria that make vitamin K, which helps our bones and prevents bleeding. The colon does need to move things through, however. Ensure that you have a minimum of one bowel movement per day to keep the colon happy and healthy.

Your Liver and Your Cholesterol

The liver has everything to do with creating and maintaining healthy cholesterol numbers. We know that cholesterol is not the bad guy we previously thought. Among other things, cholesterol is essential to making our hormones. But cholesterol does seem to be a marker of chronic low-grade inflammation that is linked with heart disease and stroke.

Here is the cholesterol story. We breathe oxygen, which in our environment is two oxygen molecules put together with a double bond. The process of respiration breaks this bond, leaving each oxygen molecule by itself. These lone molecules are called "free radicals," which can behave like a mentally unstable terrorist. Free radicals will do anything and everything to pair up again. They circulate through our bloodstream and create damage wherever they go.

Because the body knows how to heal, it sends out damage-control messages requesting help. To the rescue comes cholesterol. Cholesterol goes to the area of inflammation and creates a protective patch. The problem is that more and more free radicals are created and pass by this patch—turning the patch into lousy oxygenated cholesterol (LDL). Elevated LDL is what your doctor looks for as a marker for heart disease.

Traditional medicine treats this problem by cutting cholesterol with statin drugs. But that causes more problems. First, we need cholesterol to make our hormones. Second, a huge list of frightening side effects is associated with statin drugs. The latter doubles the risk of diabetes and increases the risk of dementia. Your cholesterol numbers are just like the red light in your car that signals when the oil is low. Turning off the light (i.e., cutting your numbers) does not fix the low-oil problem. A much more effective solution to cholesterol problems is to eliminate the free radicals that are causing the problem in the first place. We can't do anything about breathing, which creates free radicals. But there's a simple way to get rid of these critters. The answer is antioxidants, which sop up free radicals. "Great," you say. "I'll take antioxidant vitamins." Not so fast. Vitamin supplements can be a great way to naturally treat deficiencies, but your liver must deal with them just as if they were medications. An easier and more effective solution is to get your antioxidants from food. Fruits and vegetables are the best source of antioxidants.

I've had huge success with my cholesterol patients by having them do the liver cleanse, and afterward putting them on two meals a day of plant-based foods. For the third meal, they can add chicken breasts or fish to their meal. Usually people are on their own for breakfast or lunch, but they have dinner with their family. This way, they can enjoy the family meal—just take an extra helping of vegetables and skip the potatoes and grains. It's harder when you have a specialized diet that's different from everyone else's. At breakfast and lunch, we have more in our control. Most of my patients with elevated cholesterol have been able to reduce their LDL numbers an average of thirty points by doing this.

Your Liver and the Thyroid Connection

Note, too, that a liver cleanse may be the one thing you can do to increase your thyroid function. In the previous chapter, I explained that the thyroid hormone T3 is the active form and T4 is inactive (does you no good). Most of the active thyroid hormone T3 comes from the conversion of inactive T4, which occurs in the liver, and to a small degree in the kidneys. You can pour medication of inactive T4 into your body, but you won't get any active T3 and feel better unless your liver is working well. A healthy liver, along with healthy adrenal glands, will keep T3 at optimal levels. However, your liver won't have time to do its job if it's too busy and is contaminated by the chemicals in your dry-cleaned clothes and by the bisphenol A in your plastic containers. The liver message will be: "I'm busy. I have no time for thyroid hormones."

Trouble in Liver City

A liver disease called NASH (nonalcoholic steatohepatitis), or "fatty liver," is now reaching epidemic proportions in the Western world.

The translation of steatohepatitis is that our livers ("hepato") are inflamed (the "itis") and malfunctioning due to a buildup of fat ("steato"). Previously, this disease was seen only in alcoholics. Today, fatty liver is recognized as the most common cause of abnormal liver-function tests in the United States, Canada, Australia, and Europe. About one in four people in the general population now has fatty-liver disease. Because there are no early symptoms, this might be you. Fatty liver occurs when fat accumulation exceeds 5 percent of liver weight. Diet, obesity, and diabetes are among the common causes.

Does that mean that people develop fatty liver because they're fat? Yes and no. We actually don't know, because there were fat people before fatty liver became a big issue. The vast majority of people who have NASH are fat. But some thin people have NASH, too. It's just that the liver isn't functioning optimally. It isn't getting rid of what it should and is congested. It's not filtering your car.

Pharmaceutical companies are now investigating medications to treat NASH, but I've reversed the problem in all my fatty-liver patients with diet, supplements, and liver cleanses.

Remember, we're feeling this way because our hormones are not being produced and activated, due to a liver that's in trouble.

I think women are good at prevention. We're caretakers, and we're wise about health. We take our kids for checkups; we get Pap smears and mammograms. We now have to add a once-a-year or seasonal liver cleanse to our prevention list.

Be Kind

Take care of your liver, which regulates testosterone and other hormones, by reducing the toxins it must filter and doing the cleanse. A struggling liver will create hormone imbalances. It affects things you would never think of as being related to your liver, such as the inability to lose weight, elevated cholesterol, fatigue, and even, in some people, itching. My program will help restore your liver to health, improve your immune system, boost testosterone by balancing your hormones, and aid weight loss. It takes about two weeks to create a habit, and many of the liver-cleanse recommendations should become a part of your life.

A cleanse normally costs up to $900 at my clinic. I'm going to show you how to do it yourself, at home, in Chapter 7.

CHAPTER 6

Time Nutrient-Dense Eating to Lose Weight

want you to make permanent changes in your lifestyle and your attitude toward your well-being. One of the biggest shifts you implement should be eating foods that nourish your body and reduce inflammation. This dietary change (which is delicious, by the way) also melts pounds fast—without dieting. And losing weight not only makes you look great and feel better about yourself (think of the added sense of control); it also increases your testosterone levels. You're not going to convert the testosterone you have into estrogen, which is caused by body fat. In turn, of course, your testosterone helps you make more muscle instead of fat.

The best source of vitamins and minerals is food. However, most of us do not eat enough of the fruits and vegetables we need to detoxify the liver and enable it to process testosterone and other key hormones optimally. We don't eat enough plant foods to build the new cells we need and help the adrenal glands manufacture hormones at desired levels without creating inflammation in the process. In addition, the produce we do eat is less nutrient-dense than it was fifty years ago due to pollution, pesticides, farming practices, and other factors. A nonorganic salad of tomatoes, cucumbers, spinach, and peppers today delivers a fraction of the nourishment it would have back in the 1950s. I tell my patients the answer is: Eat food your great-grandmother would recognize—and eat it often through-out the day. That means eating a lot more food than you're accus-tomed to—but only the right foods.

Slim Down with Nutrients Instead of Cutting Calories

My weight-loss recommendations are based on the principle that most of us need to eat more in order to weigh less. Why? Because there are two kinds of malnourishment. There is calorie malnourish-ment, and there is nutrient malnourishment. We have an epidemic of the latter in the United States. We pack in plenty of calories and we weigh more than we need to for optimal health, but we are mal-nourished at the cellular level. That means our cells aren't working right. They don't have the ingredients they need to do their job.

Secondarily, malnourishment is a form of stress, and your body will produce and hang on to fat as a protective measure in response to stress. We have to address our nutrient malnutrition in order for our bodies to release fat. This explains why so many people have so much trouble losing weight even when they cut calories and increase exercise. Their stressed cells retain fat because they don't have the nu-trients to shed it. If you have trouble losing the weight around your middle, this is the fat that is associated with stress. Stress is also the reason that, if you take the prescription drug Prednisone, you will gain an average of six to eight pounds in one week without changing your eating or activity pattern. Prednisone stresses the adrenals by mimicking certain adrenal hormones.

The other kind of cellular stress that affects weight loss is fast-ing. Fasting, in this case, is not the one-day-without-food fast. It is any length of time that your body runs out of fuel and glucose for the brain and needs to produce it from a stress response. There are many popular diets that tell us to stick with eating two to three meals a day and forgo snacking. These diets are based on the idea that if you eat throughout the day you keep your blood sugar elevated. The truth is that most of us suffer from some degree of adrenal fatigue, and not eating for more than a few hours stresses the adrenal glands. As a result, the adrenals produce a burst of sugar from the liver. This burst is far more damaging to our weight-loss efforts than eating protein and low-glycemic fruits and vegetables—and preventing the crash in the first place. In addition, cortisol itself will increase the fat distribution around your middle.

My patient Mary Anne, fifty-eight, was a successful executive with a nonprofit organization. She worked very long hours and felt that she was relieving her stress by working out hard five days a week with a trainer. She came to me primarily to lose weight. She was very strong, but weighed 180 pounds. I focused her on increasing her intake of protein, vegetables, and fruits throughout the day—and cutting back on her workouts. It took a leap of faith for her to eat more and work out less intensely, but she had tried everything else. Within four months, she had lost thirty pounds. She was thrilled to have a routine that she could easily maintain for the rest of her life.

I've told you about the benefits of green vegetables, which are full of alkaline-rich nutrients, and the downside of sugar and processed foods, which are acidic and offer a welcoming environment for cancer cells. Bathing yourself in alkaline-rich foods increases the oxygenation of cells throughout your body and makes it really hard for cancer cells to grow. And any low-glycemic vegetable or fruit aids your weight loss.

The Skinny on Fat

Did you know that there are two ways to classify fats? Fats are known as fatty acids, and most of us have heard of monounsaturated and polyunsaturated fats. The second method of classification uses the length or size of the carbon chain in the fat molecule: short-chain fatty acids, medium-chain fatty acids, and long-chain fatty acids. The majority of fats we eat, whether from animal or plant sources, are long-chain fatty acids. Coconut oil is one of the main sources of medium-chain fatty acids in our food system and has been associated with a great deal of recent research showing its healing and anti-inflammatory properties. Because medium-chain fatty acids are smaller than long-chain fatty acids, they require less energy and fewer enzymes to break them down for digestion.

When we eat other fats, we want to make sure we're eating the right kind of fat—"good" fat like olive oil, avocados, and nuts. Walnuts, almonds, and certain other nuts are not only good for your heart and provide fiber; they also help your brain cells. Your brain actually consists mostly of fat. In the past, we assumed that nuts were fattening—and they are indeed high-calorie foods. Yet a meta-analysis of the results of thirty-one clinical studies in the June 2013 issue of the *American Journal of Clinical Nutrition* found that nuts included in subjects' diets did not boost weight, body-mass index (BMI), or waist circumference.

According to an examination of nut consumption and mortality published in 2013 in the *New England Journal of Medicine,* nuts may help you live longer, too. Researchers followed 76,464 women in the Nurses' Health Study (conducted from 1980 to 2010) and 42,498 men in the Health Professionals Follow-up Study (1986–2010). The study showed that the frequency of nut consumption was inversely associated with total and cause-specific mortality. Translation: Those who eat nuts live longer than those who do not. Remember, though, that not all nuts are created equal. One of our favorite nuts is actually not a nut but a dried seed—cashews! That's right. Technically, cashews are not nuts. They grow at the bottom of a cashew apple and are dried and eaten as a nut.

When You Eat

The time of day you eat certain foods is as important as what and how much you eat, especially if you suffer from adrenal fatigue. For example, American breakfasts set us up for a guaranteed crash in the afternoon. No "good" fat or protein is included. Everything we consume is sugary junk food or processed foods that convert to sugar. A slice of wheat bread or a bagel is a quick step toward sugar. (Yes, I said wheat bread turns into sugar and spikes your insulin.) With the first bite, a Danish or a muffin is even worse, because sugar is a main ingredient to begin with. As for cereal, read the label and see how much sugar is included, not to mention chemical preservatives. I guarantee you'll be amazed. Anything that can stay on the shelf for two years really shouldn't be labeled as food. Even if a cereal does not include added sugar, it is so processed that our bodies have to do very little work to break it down into smaller parts—which is another way of saying that it converts quickly and easily into sugar.

My favorite cereal swap is steel-cut oatmeal. We make a huge pot on the weekend, as it takes forty minutes to cook it. During the week, however, we just add what we want to a pot on the stove with some extra water—and there is our "instant" oatmeal that is low-glycemic and delicious. Add blueberries for micronutrients and walnuts for protein and good fat. That is a champion's breakfast, ready in less than five minutes.

My other favorite cereal alternative is muesli. Muesli was developed around 1900 by the Swiss physician Maximilian Bircher-Benner for patients in his hospital. It is made of dried fruits, nuts, ancient grains (my favorite), or rolled oats soaked in water or apple juice. (See my morning muesli recipe at the end of this chapter.)

The Weight-Loss Schedule

Here's how to nourish your body and eat a whole lot of food—more than you normally eat—but only foods that are loaded with vitamins, minerals, and nutrients. The malnourishment I've talked about is really a malnourishment of micronutrients. Micronutrients are the vitamins and minerals found in fruits, vegetables, beans, and other plant foods. Now, don't get me wrong. There are micronutrients in animal-based foods as well. Iron is a micronutrient, and there is plenty of iron in red meat. However, I want you to focus on getting micronutrients from plant-based foods, as these foods are low-inflammatory. You can and should eat large quantities and varieties, which makes eating more enjoyable. The fiber in plant-based foods also helps significantly in weight loss.

The cells that make up your organs and the cells that produce your hormones need micronutrients to do so. Does that mean you have to become a vegetarian? Not unless you want to. It is easier to get enough protein when you use animal-based foods in addition to plant-based foods. But you are going to eat a lot more plant foods than you have in the past. You're going to be a lot less hungry, too. Your new motto is "Eat more to weigh less."

Here's how it works:

Wake Up to Green Tea

A cup (or two or three) of caffeinated coffee in the morning after fasting all night is not nice to your adrenals. It's like waking up your adrenal glands while resting in bed, and slapping them in the face. That's not the best way to greet the day. It's jarring, although you've probably never thought of it from that perspective before. Caffeinated coffee is not a bad thing. Remember, I'm from Seattle. But most of us drink coffee in the morning on an empty stomach, before we've eaten anything else to soften the blow. Just try to stop your coffee habit, and you'll see that it's actually a drug that's addictive.

Dave Aspry, chairman of the Silicon Valley Health Institute and author of the *New York Times* bestselling book, *Bulletproof Diet*, has a way to help prevent the injury of coffee to our adrenals. Dave has created a coffee that is mold-free. (Coffee is very often contaminated with mold and has a negative effect on our hormones.) He combines this coffee with grass-fed organic butter. By drinking coffee combined with butter you do not need more than one cup and you experience no jitters and no crash. I have tried it myself and am amazed how great it tastes and how different it feels.

Ideally, drink green tea, which gives you caffeine but doesn't assault your body. Nutritionists rhapsodize about green tea, with good reason. It's full of antioxidants, which may protect us from cancer, as well as vitamin A, D, E, C, B, and more. All of these nourish your cells. If you *love* coffee, as my husband does, make sure your coffee intake is not on an empty stomach and limit your morning coffee to one cup, and then have tea after that if you still want a hot drink.

Another healthy option is to start your day with a glass of room-temperature water with the juice of half a lemon. The health benefits of doing this are significant. Lemon juice aids digestion because it is similar in atomic structure to the stomach's digestive juices. The vitamin C is also essential for gorgeous, glowing skin and is required for the synthesis of amino acids into collagen. Both collagen and connective tissue tighten and protect our skin. The lemon is also one of the most alkaline foods available. Most of us think of lemons as acidic, but the nutritional truth is that, in the body, lemon is alkaline. Bathing your cells in an alkaline environment promotes health and prevents disease. In addition, lemon juice helps cleanse the liver.

Start Your Day with Protein
Protein helps the body repair and maintain itself and is critical for the support of muscle mass. The recommended protein intake for a healthy adult is 45 to 56 grams a day. Research shows that people who choose protein for breakfast wind up eating about 200 cal-

ories less throughout the day, because this combination stabilizes blood-glucose levels and takes the edge off hunger. Forget about cereal in the morning. Switch to eggs, which contain more than 6 grams of protein each. Cook an omelet (or scramble eggs) in olive oil at a low temperature. But make sure to load up the pan with onions, spinach, tomatoes, peppers, and/or other micronutrients you've got sitting in the refrigerator. That's a perfect breakfast. If you're concerned about cholesterol, look to the studies. Research supports eggs as a good source of protein and shows that the link between eggs and cholesterol was overestimated.

Another breakfast option is nonfat plain Greek yogurt. A six-ounce container has 18 grams of protein, and you can add your own fresh fruit, like blueberries (rich in antioxidants) or apples, which have their own natural sweetness. Yogurt that already contains fruit adds "dessert" to your intake, which will cause a sugar surge and make you hungry. Add chia seeds or ground flaxseeds for a nutty taste with increased protein and good fats.

Chia seeds are rich in polyunsaturated fats, especially omega-3 fatty acids. Chia seeds' lipid profile is composed of 60 percent omega-3s, making them one of the richest plant-based sources of these fatty acids. Add seeds to foods and drinks (blended), or use them in baking. The outer layer of chia seeds swells when mixed with liquids to form a gel. The gel can be used to lower cholesterol and increase the nutrient content of foods and baked goods. To make an egg replacement, mix one tablespoon of chia seeds with three tablespoons of water and let sit for fifteen minutes.

Protein shakes and smoothies make good morning choices, too. Berries (frozen or fresh) are the basis, and you can add any other fruit you have around. One of my favorite morning smoothies combines frozen berries, an apple, a banana, one scoop of sunflower butter, and a chocolate protein mix. I combine these with coconut milk to the consistency of a milk shake. My children have no idea this is a protein shake and ask for "milk shake" in the mornings. I take fruit that is getting almost past its prime, cut it up, and put it in ziplock plastic bags in the freezer. It's ready to use when I need it. (See my vegetable-based smoothie recipe at the end of this chapter.)

If you use sandwich-size bags, you can create individual bags with a variety of fruits and empty the entire bag in the blender for a ready-to-go shake. Where does the protein come from? Some of it is contained in the fruit, and you can add more with protein mixes found in health-food stores and some grocery stores; you can also use yogurt, or even nut butters. These mixes are available in a variety of forms and flavors.

There is some debate about whether juicing is better than smoothies. Juice is like jet fuel. It hits the system and is easily absorbed with little effort. There's nothing to slow it down. If you have irritable bowel syndrome, juice is easy to digest. I prescribe juices as medicine to heal the liver's kupffer cells as part of the liver cleanse. However, juicing is difficult at cleanup time. You could argue that juices are better than smoothies, but you're less likely to make them.

Smoothies also have advantages. They are easier and quicker to prepare than juices, because you don't have as much cleaning to do. There's a health benefit because you use the whole fruit or vegetable. You get all that pulp, and the fiber is amazing. It prevents you from getting hungry an hour later, lowers cholesterol, keeps you regular, and aids weight loss. The consistency is chunkier, but you can add more liquid to create what you like. Smoothies can be mixed with coconut milk, hemp milk, almond milk, or rice milk. In the past, we were told that coconut was bad for us because we were eating the most sugary part of it, and because it is high in saturated fat. But new research has revealed the amazing health benefits of many parts of the coconut.

No, a smoothie is not as easily absorbed and readily available to the body as juice. But it is more easily absorbed than eating an apple or eating kale. Smoothies are also more affordable than juice, which requires larger quantities of ingredients. For example, it takes multiple carrots to make juice. For a smoothie, you need just one carrot, one-third of a cucumber, and a few leaves of Swiss chard or kale.

As a mother of two, who has to get two girls out the door for school in addition to getting myself ready to go to my clinic, I find that smoothies are my go-to weekday option purely because they're easier and faster. Make your own choice based on your individual preferences and needs.

Snack at Midmorning

After a protein breakfast, you probably won't feel hungry at 9:30 a.m. Yet most of us do need to eat more in order to lose weight. For a great midmorning snack, try a green smoothie or green juice as already discussed. Both are full of alkaline-rich nutrients and also help counteract the inflammatory cascade secreted by the adrenal glands. You could also have a piece of fruit or some vegetables.

A protein bar is not a good substitute. Protein bars often contain a significant amount of simple carbohydrates to which high-fructose corn syrup or chemical sweeteners have been added to make them taste good. Beware of the calorie count, too. Ideally, you should stick with real food that your body knows how to utilize and metabolize. Remember, you *can* reset your biology, and this is how you do it. The secondary, but important, overlying principle to remember when choosing your foods is to stick with fruits and vegetables that have a glycemic index of less than 50. The glycemic index assigns numerical values to different carbohydrates to indicate how fast they are converted into glucose and raise blood sugar in the body.

Lunch (No Later than 1:30 P.M.)

If you're usually starving at noon, you'll find that protein for breakfast and the midmorning snack curb that hunger. Lunch is another time to control sugar. Research tends to link eating late in general with gaining weight. A 2013 study focused on late lunch versus early lunch. In the study, which took place in Spain, where lunch is the main meal of the day, researchers followed 420 people (49.5 percent female) on a weight-loss diet for twenty weeks. Early eaters ate lunch before 3 p.m. Late eaters had the afternoon meal after 3 p.m. Early eaters lost more weight, and lost it faster, than late eaters. Interestingly, the late eaters skipped breakfast more often.

What's on the menu? How about a big salad topped with chicken breast, grilled salmon, or shrimp? Pack the salad with spinach, tomatoes, cucumbers, kale, and other greens. Or have beans, which are high in protein. Pinto beans, black beans, kidney beans, lentils, or garbanzo beans are good choices. My website, drtami.com, is full of easy nutrient-dense recipes like the one for vegetarian chili. Try to use plant protein, rather than animal protein, in at least one meal a day—and aim for two meals a day. Plant protein is much kinder to your system.

If you're a sandwich lover, that's fine, but choose only multigrain bread. What about whole wheat? It converts to sugar too fast. Whole grain has to work harder than whole wheat and other grains to convert to sugar. Make it an open-faced sandwich, using just one slice of bread. Bread is a macronutrient, and we already have way too much of that. Load your sandwich with micronutrients and protein like chicken. Sprouts are living things and great on sandwiches, as is shredded raw cabbage.

A lunch alternative with a ton of micronutrients is soup. Soup is so easy, even for the busiest woman. Just toss celery, onions, carrots, kale, or any vegetable you love into the Crock-Pot in the morning and throw in some chicken or other protein and stock. You'll have a nutrient-dense dinner waiting for you, filling your home with a delicious aroma. You can make and keep a basic stock for soup and add variations to it. If you love dessert, have fruit or yogurt with berries, although many women tell me they have no room for dessert.

Snack at 3 P.M.

This particular snack is the most crucial step to take. At 3 p.m., there's a natural dip in the way our circadian rhythms work with our adrenal glands. That's when many of us turn to sugar and/or caffeine for a pick-me-up—the worst thing to do. Instead, switch to a combination of good fats—like a small handful of walnuts, and slices of apples or pears, which contain a little natural sugar—to prevent that crash. Another favorite is cut-up veggies and hummus. This combination has the protein, natural sugars, and good fats needed at this crucial time of day.

Or start a life changer at work. Take a midafternoon "shake break," with either a protein smoothie or a veggie green smoothie. Everyone will be nicer and healthier, and the company will likely function better. Try to make the shakes at the office or bring them from home in a Mason jar, rather than buying them at a juice bar or a supermarket. They can be expensive, and provide a fraction of the nutrients you get in your homemade smoothies.

Head Off "Before Dinner" Hunger at 5 P.M.

Many people feel hungry around 5 p.m. and turn to less than optimal "easy snacks." I confess that cheese and crackers was my own downfall until I changed my ways. To help my two daughters stave off hunger pangs before dinner, I make a big plate of celery, cauliflower, carrots, broccoli, and other veggies with hummus or another dip on the side. I put it out for my daughters and don't have to worry whether they eat their vegetables at dinner. They already had vegetables. Try it yourself to increase your micronutrient intake. Hummus is just chickpeas and tahini, and you can add nonfat yogurt to make it creamier. (See page 140 for a wonderful hummus recipe.)

Dinner by 6:30 P.M.

This is what your evening meal looks like: There's a hierarchy of protein: Fish is better than chicken, and chicken or turkey is better than red meat. Plan on three and a half ounces of lean protein. Accompany the protein with two bright-colored vegetables like yam, broccoli, or eggplant. This is in addition to your salad. If you really love your starches, add pasta or other simple carbohydrates, like brown rice, in a portion size comparable to the inside of your palm or a tennis ball. However, for the thirty days of my program, I want you to avoid these simple starches and carbohydrates.

If you're going to eat red meat, understand the difference between grass-fed beef and regular beef. In the latter case, cattle are fed corn to fatten them up. The corn diet creates streaks of fat in the beef—saturated fat, which is bad for you. It is done to make the cows get fat fast, which is good for business. Grass-fed beef has less saturated fat. However, it's not easy to get the real thing. The meat industry can feed grass to the cows only a portion of the time and legally claim that the animals are grass-fed, although they're also fed corn. Look for "grass fed, grass finished" beef to get the real thing, which has much less saturated fat.

Because eating healthy is a challenge, one tip for getting better animal protein is to use the Internet to find a farmer who will ship to your area. Get your friends and neighbors to share in the purchase of a side of beef. You'll be supporting small farmers, eating healthier, and connecting with friends and neighbors at the same time. Another option is to order seafood or organic grass-fed beef online from Vital Choice. It has truly delicious options, delivered to your home.

You can also eat high-protein beans for the evening meal— or quinoa, a high-protein ancient grain that is full of vitamins and minerals. The Food and Agriculture Organization (FAO) of the United Nations declared 2013 "The International Year of Quinoa." People sometimes have trouble finding recipes for quinoa, but there are now cookbooks devoted to it, and you can find recipes online. Many restaurants also include quinoa on the menu these days.

Many people with adrenal fatigue need a snack before bed. If you have trouble sleeping and want a snack at night, you can have some Greek yogurt with blueberries or an apple with almond butter. Otherwise, there is no evening snack. At night our bodies slow down, and it's not a good time for digestion. Listen to your body and learn the difference between hunger and craving. In Chapter 10, you'll learn about specific supplements to help with various types of food cravings that plague us.

What about sweeteners? Stevia (rebaudiana), which comes from the leaf of a South American plant, is best. It's much sweeter than sugar and is FDA-approved. Although Truvia, a manufactured sugar substitute, is sometimes confused with stevia, it is not the same. Truvia has three ingredients: erythritol, Rebiana, and natural flavors. Never use aspartame or other artificial sweeteners, which screw up your hormones. I often serve this fun dessert: I cut up some apples,

THE KEFIR STORY

Kefir is a dairy drink that contains a wide range of vitamins, minerals, and a variety of probiotic organisms (similar to the organisms found in yogurt) that live symbiotically in our bodies and create a huge health benefit. Probiotics help our immune system as well as prevent and treat constipation and diarrhea. At Children's Hospital here in Seattle, we give probiotics to children who have eczema, because it helps with immunity issues and treats diarrhea. Did you know that your gut also creates one-third of the brain chemicals that affect brain function? We often say, "I have a gut feeling" about something. It's because we do. The gut literally makes neurotransmitters for the brain. If your gut isn't healthy, you're not going to think well. Studies also show that kefir has antibacterial and antifungal properties. However, stress, cortisol, hormone imbalance, and lack of sleep cause the body to become more acidic, and an acidic environment kills probiotics.

Drinking kefir is a way to restore and replenish a population of these organisms. Kefir is derived from the Turkish word *keif,* which

add stevia and cinnamon, and bake it in the oven until the apples are slightly soft—about twenty minutes. It tastes like apple pie, and my family loves it.

Prepare in Advance

When I get home from grocery shopping, I don't put the fruits and vegetables in the refrigerator immediately. I wash them off, cut them up right away, and divide them among plastic sandwich bags. Our bodies are designed to seek the easy way, which is part of the reason we

translates to the phrase "good feeling." Cultures around the world have attributed healing powers to it. The fermented-milk product originated centuries ago in the Caucasus and is made from the milk of cows, goats, or sheep. It's slightly sour due to the activity of the symbiotic bacteria and tastes like a yogurt drink. The nice thing is that kefir, which contains a host of beneficial microbes, has been touted as one of the most potent probiotic foods available.

We need vitamin K, which is lacking in the American diet, to build bone. Vitamin K is a product of the bacterial fermentation in our gut. It's found in dark-green vegetables, such as kale, spinach, Brussels sprouts, Swiss chard, green beans, asparagus, broccoli, mustard greens, turnip greens, collard greens, thyme, romaine lettuce, sage, oregano, cabbage, celery, sea vegetables, cucumbers, and leeks, as well as in cauliflower, tomatoes, and blueberries.

Because there is only a small amount of vitamin K in the foods that contain it, it's very hard to get enough of it without taking a supplement. But we believe kefir may be a good source of K, which is very important for women who are entering hormone-deficiency stages. Kefir is also high in calcium and phosphorus.

like packaged, processed foods. Make it convenient to choose wisely. At my house, we grab the cut-up veggie bags when we head out as a family on our way to soccer, figure skating, or dance classes. I pop them into our lunches and reach for them when I open the fridge and start "just looking." The goal is to have the food staring back at you be something other than leftover pizza, cherry pie, or a quart of ice cream.

Allergies and Weight

Some women, such as my patient Laura, have more serious problems with losing weight than the rest of us. Laura was five-six and weighed about 210 pounds. At her first appointment with me, she announced, "I'm not someone who goes to the drive-thru and orders three Big Macs. Yes, I obviously eat more than my body needs, but not to the degree my weight suggests. I've had my thyroid checked, and there's nothing wrong. Yet I just can't get the weight off."

I immediately suspected stress, inflammation, or food allergies. It's very hard to lose weight if you have a food allergy, because your body can easily absorb only sugar and simple carbohydrates, and these are fattening. I tried allergy tests first. The results showed that Laura was allergic to eggs—specifically, egg whites. Ironically, she ate egg whites every morning, thinking they were much healthier than the whole egg. The first step was to eliminate eggs from her diet, which isn't easy, because there are eggs in anything that's baked and can stay on a shelf in this country. I put her on a regimen of fresh vegetables, protein, and whole grains like quinoa and farro, as well as a program to heal inflammation in her gut. The program included two supplements and probiotics. For extra help, I added chewable digestive enzymes, which allowed her to digest and absorb nutrients more easily, and gave her gut time to heal.

Laura was determined to stick to my recommendations. She proceeded to lose thirty pounds in six months, simply by changing her way of eating and respecting her customized sensitivities. For the first time in her life, she was able to lose more than ten pounds—and she did it without going on a diet. The point is, not everything (including a seemingly benign food like egg whites) is a good idea for every single person. Penicillin saves lives, but it can also kill people who are allergic to it.

There are actually two types of food allergies that I discuss with patients at my clinic: IgA cells are immune cells in our bodies that protect us, and IgA-mediated food allergies show up immediately after you eat a particular food. You eat a peanut and instantly can't breathe. The other type of food allergy involves a delayed immune response. You eat green beans, and three days later you have joint pain and a migraine headache. This is due to inflammation. Because the inflammation can go anywhere the blood goes, it can also cause fatigue and acne. Due to the inflammation in the gut, sugar and carbohydrates quickly get absorbed with no problem. But the body still isn't satisfied, as it needs the building blocks to make cells like amino acids, plus vitamins and minerals. If our cells don't absorb these important nutrients, they can send the message that they need more, causing hunger and overeating.

In my practice, I have evaluated thousands of patients for food sensitivities and allergies, and I am always surprised by the results. This is truly a case of one size does *not* fit all. Many patients tell me that they believe they are gluten-intolerant. I tell them maybe. And there is a test to check for that. Many people feel better steering clear of gluten for various reasons, and I support focusing on protein, vegetables, and fruits. Fortunately, you don't need a doctor to eliminate a food allergy. You can order tests yourself to determine whether you're allergic (and to what) by submitting a blood sample through the mail to a lab, such as www.saveonlabs.com or on drtami.com. When you avoid foods to which you're sensitive, your gut lining can heal. Eventually, your body can start absorbing amino acids, rather than just the sugar and simple carbohydrates that stop you from losing weight.

Other Barriers to Weight Loss

We eat while we are distracted. We eat when we're standing, while working, and in our cars. We drink gallons of coffee without even realizing it. Basically, we don't eat with intention. What does that mean? It means sitting down, being present as you dine, saturating your taste buds, and enjoying a meal. I think that's why we're always searching for more to eat. We don't experience flavor and satisfaction, and sometimes we don't even realize we've eaten all that we have. And we certainly don't get the nutrition we need. Digestion actually starts with the look and the smell of food, which leads the brain to release chemicals in your saliva that start the digestion process. But we don't look and smell and savor. You can change that and make it matter. If you do, you'll realize that even your work is more successful because each thing you do is intentional.

Quick Course in Smoothies

Green smoothies are a great way to increase the amount of micronutrients you eat. Smoothies have the added benefit of being easier and quicker than juicing (though I am a big fan of juicing, too), and they have all the fiber found in vegetables and fruits. The fiber is itself a treatment for high cholesterol and high blood pressure.

How to start:

1. Purchase a blender that will puree vegetables. Vitamix, Ninja, and Magic Bullet are a few names. These do not have to be expensive.
2. Add a liquid when you make smoothies. You need coconut water or milk or one of the other liquids I mentioned earlier, because otherwise the consistency will be like sludge.
3. Start with green. Green vegetables are magic. Choose any green you like. Some of my favorites are kale, Swiss chard, rainbow chard, beet tops, arugula, and spinach. I put one leaf of several of the above

in my morning smoothie. I also add about a two-inch piece of cucumber and a stalk of celery. You can add one carrot and one piece of fruit. If you have problems with prediabetes or diabetes, or want to lose weight, choose a fruit with a low-glycemic index, such as an apple or a pear. Add coconut water, which is not sugary and is also fat-free. It's a superfluid and contains the potassium of more than four bananas. Everyone with high blood pressure needs potassium. One ounce of unflavored coconut water contains 5.45 calories. It doesn't have to be refrigerated, and it's available in large containers that you can store on a shelf for long periods of time.

4. Consider options for spicing up your smoothies: Add a thumbnail piece of ginger, one-fourth of a beet, and/or chia seeds. You can even add peppers to really spice it up.

5. Try a cold green smoothie. That's how I prefer mine. I pour the mixture over ice or blend it with ice, and often serve it in a wineglass. It makes me feel special. I use a Mason jar if I take a smoothie "on the go," as I bring my girls to school or get to work. I also use the jars to store extra smoothies.

Fill the jar to the top to decrease the amount of air (and the oxidation process that occurs when fruits and vegetables are left out). Ever notice how an apple turns brown when exposed to the air? That's oxidation, and it's not good for us or for the apple. The remainder of the smoothie can be consumed when you return home at the end of the day and are hungry. Ideally, it should not be kept in the fridge for more than twenty-four hours. Fresh is best, to benefit from all the nutrients.

DR. TAMI'S MORNING MUESLI

- 1 cup ancient grain mix (You can use rolled oats.)
- ½ cup raw nuts (My favorite are almonds, followed by hazelnuts.)
- ½ cup shredded unsweetened coconut
- ⅓ cup sunflower seeds
- ⅓ cup pumpkin seeds
- ⅓ cup chia seeds (optional for a thicker consistency)
- 2 teaspoons cinnamon

Mix all the ingredients in a bowl, and store in a large glass jar.

When you are ready to eat, prepare this way:

Put 1 to 2 cups of the mixture into a bowl. Cover with unsweetened apple juice and one apple grated (leave peel on). Mix with organic nonfat Greek yogurt to the consistency you like. You can eat this right away, but I like it left overnight.

ALMOND MILK

For great-tasting smoothies, almond milk is an alternative to coconut water or coconut milk, and it has the added bonus of being protein-rich.

You will need:

- Organic raw almonds
- Water
- Bowl
- Measuring cup
- Strainer
- Blender or food processor
- Cheesecloth or fine-mesh nut bag

Cover the almonds with water to an inch above the almonds, which will soak up the water.

Soak overnight or up to two days. The longer you soak the almonds, the creamier your almond milk will be. Drain and rinse the almonds with cool running water. The almonds should feel slightly squishy.

Combine the almonds with 2 cups of water in a blender or food processor. This will give you almond milk that is the consistency of 2 percent milk. If you prefer the experience of drinking fat-free milk, use more water.

Pulse the almond-water mixture to separate the almonds and then blend on high for 2 to 3 minutes. You may need to scrape the sides as you go. If you are using a food processor, blend for 4 minutes, using a spatula in between to scrape down the sides.

Line the strainer with cheesecloth or a nut bag, and place the nut mixture in the strainer. You may need to do this in batches, depending on the size of your strainer.

Gather the edges of the cheesecloth and twist closed, or close the nut bag. Squeeze out the almond milk through the cloth. Pour and enjoy, or place in Mason jars for up to two days.

Use the leftover almond meal in oatmeal, muffins, or smoothies. Try one teaspoon of vanilla or cinnamon or honey—or all three— for variations. If you prefer step-by-step video instructions, go to drtami.com (under "recipes") for a video format.

PAPA'S TRADITIONAL HUMMUS

This fabulous recipe, provided by Sonya Khazaal, of Seattle's award-winning restaurant Phoenecia, is great for the liver cleanse, and for healing the adrenal glands, and truly feeds the spirit:

You will need:

- 1½ cups chickpeas (garbanzo beans)
- The night before, soak the chickpeas in plenty of cold water (completely covering them with an inch of water above). In the morning, discard the water, rinse the chickpeas, and you're all set.
- 2 teaspoons salt
- 2 garlic cloves, or 1 teaspoon garlic powder
- ¾ cup tahini
- ½ cup lemon juice
- ¼ teaspoon cayenne pepper
- 2 tablespoons parsley, for garnish
- Olive oil, for garnish

Drain the chickpeas and place them in a pot with about three times their amount of water and a teaspoon of salt.

Boil vigorously for 10 minutes, then turn down the heat and cover the pot.

Simmer for 1 hour, or until the chickpeas are very soft.

Drain and keep the water for use in a later step.

Set aside ½ cup of the chickpeas for a garnish, a nice traditional touch.

Place the remaining chickpeas in a food processor.

Crush the garlic with 1 teaspoon of salt, then add this to the food processor.

Slowly add the tahini and the lemon juice. Add a little of one, followed by a little of the other, until you have used all you have. Blend in a little of the water you set aside from boiling the chickpeas. Adjust the salt and lemon juice to taste.

Serve on a platter with hummus spread thin and garnish with a little cayenne, parsley, olive oil, and the ½ cup chickpeas you set aside.

Enjoy!

As you can see, you have many different food choices, and the idea is not to feel deprived and to feed your cells. Diets don't work, but changing your routines and your relationship to food does.

PART THREE

The 30-Day Plan (and Beyond)

Can you spare a month to lose eight to ten pounds without dieting, clear brain fog, look younger, sleep better, and be happier and healthier? You can take control with my three-part action plan to change your life.

Detox, Heal, Rebalance— Safely and Effectively

Part I (Days 1–15): The Liver Cleanse
This metabolic cleanse restores your liver to health so that it can process your hormones, such as testosterone, estrogen, and progesterone, in top form. Most people have a dysfunctional liver and don't realize it. They have no clue, because there are no symptoms. The liver cleanse will energize your life by cleaning out the filter, which is clogged with all you have eaten, breathed, and absorbed, knowingly and not.

Part II (Days 16–30): Adrenal Healing
This segment starts your adrenal glands on the path to healing. It takes robust adrenals to supply you with the hormones you need for a better body, brain, bones, and skin.

Part III (Days 16–30, Concurrently with Adrenal Healing): Resetting Hormones
In this section, you'll address your individual hormone deficiencies and imbalances, using specific over-the-counter herbs, vitamins/

minerals, and supplements as medications—without the side effects of drugs. These nonprescription products boost levels of testosterone and other essential hormones (or reduce them when necessary).

My recommendations are based on clinical experience with patients, plus my review of studies in the literature. I will also educate you in the use of foods, if any, that can boost and balance each hormone. I'll provide meditation instructions and other exercises that will increase your hormones as well as your overall health.

You're going to change the way you eat, move, think, and supplement—all within thirty days—to look and feel your best as long as you live.

CHAPTER 7

Part I: The Liver Cleanse

(Days 1–15)

To begin removal of toxins from your liver:

✧ Limit foods to choices not processed by the liver.
✧ Avoid foods that overburden the liver.
✧ Do a body scrub daily.
✧ Use a sauna, if possible.
✧ Supplement with herbs and vitamins/minerals.
✧ Move, stretch, and get out into sunlight.
✧ Start *now*.

My plan starts with the fifteen-day liver cleanse because the doctor in me worries about both your safety and your success. I don't want you to get superexcited and jump right in to boost your hormones until your liver is squeaky-clean. For most of us, our liver "machinery" is too clogged with grime and toxins to operate properly. You want to turn the place into a streamlined, superefficient factory. But you have to clean it up first to ensure that the rest of your efforts on the 30-Day Plan will be successful. However, the cleanse requires some prioritizing. You may think, "Oh, I'll skip the liver part. I'll do it later." That attitude will sabotage the results.

There's no way a struggling liver can activate testosterone and other hormones or remove fat and cholesterol from your body. If you don't take care of your liver, your hormones will only be partially metabolized and detoxified. This leaves them more dangerous and active than they were originally. Your body can make carcinogenic metabolites out of your hormones. My cleanse pulls out all the toxins that have piled up in your liver and disposes of them. Don't worry. This is not one of those torturous cleanses that restricts you to drinking lemon water and vegetable juice. Instead, this is a comprehensive nutrition, supplement, and detoxification system that does more than clean out the gunk. This detox is an essential first step in boosting and balancing testosterone.

Nutrition Guidelines

Because the detox process is work for the liver, it's important not to add to it. That's why you now follow the "Foods to Include" part of the chart on pages 150–151. These are foods that aren't processed by the liver and, in effect, give your liver a vacation. You also want to eliminate items that interfere with the Phase 1 or Phase 2 detox systems. See the "Foods to Avoid" part of the chart.

Eat as many (and as much) of the "Foods to Include" items as you wish. This is not about deprivation; it's about abundance. I believe it's much easier to be successful if you replace, rather than simply remove, unhealthy options. Remember, this is not a "diet." I want you to eat three meals a day, plus two snacks of nutrient-dense vegetables and fruits.

Daily Food Schedule

1. Drink detoxification tea when you wake in the morning. Green tea or herbal tea can be substituted, but detox tea is a much better option. Drink detoxification tea as often as you like—the more the better. The entire purpose of Phase 1 detoxification of the liver is to make toxins more water-soluble and therefore easier for the body to eliminate. The tea ensures that you urinate those toxins out. (Yes, you'll make lots of trips to the bathroom.) I offer a specific detoxification tea to my patients, but you can find detox teas in many supermarkets, health-food stores, and online. Just enter "detox tea" in your search engine and a large array of options will appear. Look on store shelves for teas labeled "detox tea"—or for teas with one or more of the following ingredients: licorice root, cinnamon, juniper berry, dandelion, burdock.

2. Eat protein for breakfast. Ideally, start the day with a protein shake. I prefer the one called MediClear or the one I created, because it offers detoxification benefits in addition to the protein you need in the morning. (Eggs are on the liver-cleanse "Avoid" list.) You can buy MediClear, which I want you to drink once or twice a day, over the counter or online. It draws out toxins from the liver, and tastes great mixed with berries and coconut milk, almond milk, or hemp milk (unsweetened, of course). If you want more than a shake, add steel-cut oatmeal with blueberries, which is very filling, to your breakfast.

3. Have a midmorning snack (around 10:30 a.m.). Select from low-glycemic vegetables or fruits on the approved list on the next page. Or you can substitute the shake if you haven't had it for breakfast.

4. Eat lunch (ideally by 1:30 p.m.). This should consist of lean protein (choose from the approved list), with more veggies.

5. Have a midafternoon snack (before 3 p.m.). Low-glycemic vegetables or fruits on the approved list will satisfy you.

6. Eat dinner by 6:30 p.m. if possible. The meal must include protein from the approved list, two brightly colored vegetables, and a salad.

I also want you to drink two to four glasses of fresh organic vegetable juices or green smoothies a day to bathe your liver cells (called kupffer cells) in nutrients. These cells destroy bacteria and worn-out blood cells. Or use the juices for your midmorning or afternoon snack. For example, cucumber, celery, kale, carrots, apples, and organic coconut water can be churned up to the consistency you want for a liver-friendly midmorning smoothie snack. Magic Bullet or Nutri-Bullet food processors are inexpensive machines to start off with.

Liver Cleanse

FOODS TO INCLUDE	FOODS TO AVOID
Apples, apricots, avocado, bananas, blueberries, cherries, grapes, kiwis, mangoes, melons, nectarines, papaya, peaches, pears, pineapples, plums, prunes, raspberries, strawberries. Fresh is best, or unsweetened frozen.	Grapefruit, sweetened fruits (canned or frozen) and fruit juices, corn, tomatoes, tomato sauce, creamed vegetables, gluten-containing products, including wheat, spelt, kamut, barley, rye.
	Soybeans, tofu, tempeh, soy milk, soy sauce, any product containing soy protein, peanuts, peanut butter.
Artichokes, arugula, asparagus, bean sprouts, bell peppers, bok choy, broccoli, Brussels sprouts, cabbage, cauliflower, celery, cucumbers, eggplants, endive, escarole, green beans, green peas, jicamas, lettuce, mushrooms, okras, radishes, spinach, squash (summer and winter), sweet potatoes, taros, turnips, yams, zucchinis. All fresh, raw, steamed, grilled, sautéed, roasted, or juiced.	Tuna, swordfish, shellfish, beef, pork, cold cuts, hot dogs, sausages, canned meats.
	Milk, cheese, eggs, cream, butter, yogurt, ice cream, nondairy creamers. Margarine, butter, shortening, processed or hydrogenated oil, peanut oil, mayonnaise. Coconut and olive oil are good alternatives.
Rice (white, brown, sushi, wild), oats (gluten-free), quinoa, millet, amaranth, buckwheat. Products made from rice.	Soda and soft drinks (including sugar-free), alcoholic beverages, coffee, black tea.
Legumes, including peas and lentils (except soybeans). Nuts (except peanuts): almonds, cashews, macadamia,	

walnuts, pumpkin seeds, brazil nuts, sunflower seeds —whole or as nut butter.

White or brown sugar, corn syrup, honey. Chocolate, ketchup, relish, BBQ sauce, chutney, other condiments.

All fresh or frozen fish (except shellfish), such as salmon, halibut, sole, mahimahi, cod, snapper, etc. Wild is better than farm-raised fish. Chicken, turkey, lamb, and wild game (venison, buffalo, elk, etc.). Organic and hormone-free is always best.

Milk substitutes, such as rice milk, oat milk, almond or other nut milk, and egg substitutes. Cold-pressed oils such as olive oil, flaxseed, canola, safflower, sunflower, sesame, walnut, hazelnut, or pumpkin seed.

Filtered or distilled water, mineral water, decaffeinated tea, green tea, herbal tea. Chicory syrup, stevia, blackstrap molasses, fruit sweeteners, such as Lo Han fruit, pure maple syrup, yacon syrup. Vinegars (except grain source), wasabi, mustard, horseradish, pesto (cheese-free), and all spices.

Some of the foods on the "Avoid" list are acidic, which means that they provide a welcoming environment for cancer cells to grow. Certain other items on the "Avoid" list, such as tomatoes, are perfectly healthy, but they are processed by the liver. We want the liver to recuperate for these two weeks. Yes, you must give up wine and other alcohol temporarily in order to give the liver a rest, let it do its job, and increase its capacity to deal with all the toxins it must eliminate.

The liver detoxification system consists of two parts: Phase 1 and Phase 2. Foods and medications can either activate these systems or hinder their function. Did you know that grapefruit slows down the Phase 1 cytochrome P450 detox system by approximately 30 percent? This means that eating grapefruit can cause toxins to build up in the liver. Worse, medications you rely on may not be activated and may actually be ineffective! That's why your doctor tells you not to eat grapefruit with some drugs. You want to focus on foods that support and promote the Phase 1 and 2 detoxification—those on my "Foods to Include" list.

Typically, people lose weight during the cleanse because they don't eat bread, pasta, sugar, alcohol, or processed foods. You are going to shed pounds automatically without such foods—and by increasing your liver's ability to remove fat. Fats in your body have to pass through your liver and be disposed of. In my experience with thousands of patients, a liver detox makes all these efforts more successful.

It's sometimes easier to give things up for a cleanse than for a diet. The hardest part for most people is eating out during the cleanse. Tell the waiter, "Please hold the bread." Bread is hard to resist if you go to a restaurant when you're hungry.

The Juicing Commitment

Juicing during the liver cleanse is like taking medication to treat your liver. Juicing is preferable to smoothies in the liver cleanse process, because smoothies are harder for the body to absorb. But do what's feasible for you. Remember that even doing 10 percent is so much better than nothing. Just keep your expectations about what you get out of the cleanse in line with how much you put into it. Too many women take an "all or nothing" approach. If they can't do the cleanse perfectly, they drop it entirely. Practice the art of grace with yourself—and prepare in advance in order to be the most successful.

Drink organic vegetable juices you make yourself. Juicing is hard, timewise. It takes planning and effort, but it's like jet fuel for your cells. I tell my patients, "You have to make the commitment and do it." Green juices are an amazing, easy-to-absorb, nutrient-dense food, and do not require processing by the liver. If there is such a thing as "healthy candy," green juices are it. They are also alkaline and don't encourage cancer cells and inflammation to thrive.

If you buy packaged juices, note that the pasteurization process kills all the good nutrients, as well as harmful bacteria. That process also kills the living energetic plant enzymes that do the very work you're drinking the juices for. Check out the glycemic indexes of some of the bottled or canned juices. You'll see that they have so much sugar that you might as well eat a doughnut. For example, an eight-ounce serving of V8 juice has 8 grams of sugar per eight-ounce serving.

However, some people who have severe time constraints feel that it's worth the investment to find places that make fresh organic vegetable juices while you wait. In Seattle, you can actually order these juices through AmazonFresh and get them delivered to your door.

In New York, juice bars have opened everywhere, including at some health clubs. You can order fresh juice and stand there while it's made right in front of you. It's expensive, but guess what? Many things in life are a trade-off of time versus money. If you want to fly from Seattle to New York and you don't mind two stopovers and an eleven-hour trip, you can book a cheaper flight. If you don't have the time, you're going to pay more money for a direct flight. You just have to figure out whether the trade-off is worth it to you.

When one of my patients and her husband were doing the liver cleanse together, she told me, "Oh, we so do not have time for the juicing." I gave her the names of three local companies that make fresh organic juices. The next time I saw her, I asked, "How did it go?" She said, "I couldn't believe how expensive it was. All of a sudden, I felt that making the juice had a real value. So I made time to do it." She said, "Now I keep a dollar sign in my mind, to remind me how much value I'm providing to my family. I know it's weird, but I feel it's worth it." Maintaining your house or apartment is a similar example. Do you clean the house yourself? Or is it worth it to you to pay someone else to do it?

Ideally, I want you to drink twelve to sixteen ounces of green juice, divided, during the day, or all at once. But if you can only manage two smoothies, don't "should" yourself. Celebrate whatever level of success you can manage given where you are right now.

Body Treatments

Once a day during the cleanse, do a dry body scrub using a scrubbing mitt and Himalayan salt (available at health-food stores) before showering or bathing. The scrub stimulates the lymphatic system and helps with exfoliation. Your skin absorbs toxins and chemicals, and dry-brushing helps the skin's detoxification abilities.

My patients also benefit from a sauna at a spa, health club, or gym. Saunas stimulate Phase 2 detox because you sweat out toxins. A tradition in Finland, saunas date back more than two thousand years, according to some researchers, and Finns credit their endurance and longevity to the sauna custom. What happens to your body during a sauna? Your metabolism and your pulse rate increase, your blood vessels grow more flexible, and your extremities benefit from increased circulation. Some enthusiasts report feeling peace and contentment, as well as physical rejuvenation, after spending time in a sauna. Many swear by its power to relieve the symptoms of colds and other minor illnesses, revive muscles after tough exertion, and even clear the complexion.

Stay in the sauna only as long as you feel comfortable, increasing the time with each visit. Feelings of light-headedness or dizziness are signs that you should get out. Be sure that you drink plenty of water, too, because you'll be sweating buckets. If you can, enjoy a sauna daily during the liver cleanse. If you have a heart condition, however, check with your doctor before starting to use a sauna. Not every gym or health club has a sauna, but it's worth asking about.

We women don't like to perspire. We think it's unfeminine. But real women do sweat. Sweating draws out all those toxins and brings circulation to your skin surface. Anytime you increase circulation, you "feed" your body. And remember, you do take a shower afterward. Anything that makes you sweat is good for your liver. We're supposed to sweat, and we're designed to do it. Ballet dancers' skin glows when they sweat.

Supplements for the Liver Cleanse

The liver-friendly food plan and body scrubs are necessary for a successful detox, but they can't do it all. Herbs, vitamins/minerals, and other supplements have a role to play as well. They specifically aid the detox process through the Phase 1 and Phase 2 system—and help heal the liver's kupffer cells. These over-the-counter products don't need to be taken long-term—just for the fifteen days of this cleanse. Ideally, you will cleanse once a season, as I do myself. If the liver is too overwhelmed to eliminate all the toxins on its "to do" list, the remaining toxins get stuck in your body.

For the Fifteen-Day Cleanse, take:

- **Protein Shake:** 1–2 glasses per day of MediClear or the protein that I created for my liver cleanse. Both are available at drtami. com.
- **Multivitamin:** 1 daily. The liver needs enough vitamin C, B1, B5, and B12, selenium, zinc, and magnesium. A good multivitamin, such as Nutreince (Calton Nutrition) or Ultra Preventive (Douglas Laboratories), will provide you with what you need.
- **Phosphatidylcholine:** 100 mg twice a day
- **Milk Thistle:** 100–200 mg twice a day
- **Fenugreek:** 400 mg daily
- **Slippery Elm:** 600 mg daily

The entire cleanse kit can be found at drtami.com to save you time in finding it at all. I have created the above in a convenient pack to make life easier.

Lifestyle

Get 20 to 30 minutes of light exercise in the form of walking or riding a bike every day.

Get 20 minutes of outside light daily.

Stretch daily. (You can stretch your calves while you brush your teeth.)

Take Care of Yourself During the Cleanse

On Days 2–3, you're going to feel yucky, because your body is releasing lots of toxins into your bloodstream. The more toxins you have, the worse you're going to feel. Yay! They're leaving your body and ridding it of disease.

You may feel fatigued or as if you have a cold coming on. If you feel tired, go to bed early. Take a nap. Don't underestimate the demands on your body during the cleanse. Just because the effort is not external, such as moving out of your house and into a new one (or running a marathon), doesn't mean it won't consume a huge amount of energy. Respect that and take care. This is your time to focus on yourself. If you don't, you're no good to anybody else. Don't fall into the trap of putting yourself last.

When to Start

Everyone needs a liver cleanse once a year. If you take medications on a regular basis, just want to be the healthiest you can be, or travel a lot, do a liver cleanse once each season. What's the travel connection? Airports are stressful, and cortisol zooms when you're there, even if your baggage doesn't get lost and there are no delays caused by the weather. Once you're on a plane, you're also exposed to more pollutants and are usually less in control of your food choices.

As I said in Chapter 5, my favorite time to do my own liver detox is before the holidays. I call it my pre-tox. Studies show that people make fewer bad decisions about food, beverages, and exercise when they do a pre-holidays cleanse, because they don't want to ruin the results at Thanksgiving, Christmas, and New Year's events.

But the very best time to do your first cleanse is NOW. Don't wait for the "perfect" time. There is no such thing. Jump in and do the best you can to improve your health today. The success of the cleanse depends on how closely you adhere to the regimen, but any effort is an improvement.

However, if you're sick and taking antibiotics, wait until you're well again to start the cleanse. It's one of the wonders of modern medicine that you can take an antibiotic when you have an infection and recover. But that's not a good time to do a liver cleanse. Your body needs all its resources at this time.

You're on Your Way

Once you've detoxed your liver, you have a clean slate. Now your liver can activate testosterone, as well as estrogen and progesterone. The liver can process these hormones and prepare them biologically to go to work—in the exact, correct amounts. Remember, testosterone is the secret hormone that fills you with energy, improves brain function, increases libido, makes weight loss faster and easier, protects your bones, and guards against breast cancer and even endometrial cancer. My cleanse allows the liver to boost the amount of active testosterone in your body without actually increasing the total quantity of testosterone. That means more benefits without side effects.

CHAPTER 8

Part II: Adrenal Repair

(Days 16–30)

To start healing and boosting your adrenal glands:

✧ Eat adrenal-friendly, mostly alkaline, low-glycemic foods.
✧ Continue the same daily food schedule outlined on pages 149–150 of the liver cleanse.
✧ Use healing herbs, vitamins/minerals, and adrenal extracts.
✧ Manage stress and improve sleep.
✧ Belly-breathe and meditate.

Now that you've completed the liver cleanse, you're ready to heal and to boost your adrenal glands. The adrenals are another "factory" in the body—your own manufacturing plant for testosterone and other hormones.

Refer back to the adrenal self-test you took on page 91, which gives you a good idea of whether you've got adrenal fatigue. How did you score? If you do have this condition, the adrenals can't produce the levels of hormones you need to feel and look your best. These glands are too pooped to perform. They need tender loving care to heal and return to full operating capacity. Even if your adrenals haven't reached the point of fatigue, they can still use help in maintaining optimal function.

My adrenal-healing segment is part of the journey to hormone health, and specifically boosts your testosterone levels naturally. It sets you up to supply the adrenals with micronutrients and alkaline nourishment, and to address the stress that diminishes adrenal performance.

Nutrition for Healing the Adrenals

The liver-friendly foods you've been eating since Day 1 of the 30-Day Plan are mostly adrenal-friendly, too, and have already started to heal your adrenal glands. However, at Day 16, the menu shifts to an entirely adrenal-focused food selection. Nutrition can have a significantly powerful effect on your adrenals. Food is fuel for your body, but it is also information. For example, you need fats for adrenal healing—and salt is okay. A craving for salt is common among adrenal-fatigue patients. As for concerns about salt and hypertension, research shows that salt affects the blood pressure of only a minority of people.

Adrenals and the Sugar Blues

The adrenal hormone cortisol helps keep blood sugars steady to free your day from excessive highs and lows. The adrenals often can't keep up with this important task when taxed by your go-go lifestyle. Remember, when you eat is just as important as what you eat. Some popular diets encourage you not to snack, which is the very worst thing you can do for your adrenal glands. Cutting out snacks causes a drop in blood sugar, which in itself is a stress. The adrenals must also work harder to produce more cortisol to raise your blood sugar. Double zowie!

What to Eat

The perfect adrenal (and hormone) diet is composed of good-quality protein, such as fish, chicken, and eggs, and plant-based foods like

legumes, beans, seeds, and nuts, plus low-glycemic fruits and vegetables, and good fats. A small amount of dairy is okay. However, if
your goal is to lose more weight, avoiding dairy products during the
second half of the 30-Day Plan will make you more successful. See
the food chart below for good choices.

Common Alkaline Foods Good for the Adrenals

VEGETABLES	FRUITS	PROTEIN	MISCELLANEOUS
Asparagus	Apples	Beans	Apple cider vinegar
Beets	Apricots	Chicken breast	Cinnamon, curry, ginger
Broccoli	Avocados	Eggs	Fresh vegetable juice
Brussels sprouts	Bananas	Flaxseeds	Green juices
Cabbage	Berries	Goat milk	Mineral water
Carrots	Cantaloupes	Kefir	Stevia sweetener
Cauliflower	Cherries	Nuts	Teas: ginseng, herbal, kombucha
Chard	Figs	Pumpkin seeds	
Collard greens	Grapefruits	Sesame seeds	
Cucumbers	Grapes	Sunflower seeds	
Dandelions	Honeydews	Tofu	
Eggplants	Lemons	Yogurt	
Kale	Limes		
Kohlrabi	Nectarines		
Lettuce	Oranges		
Mushrooms	Peaches		
Mustard greens	Pears		
Onions	Pineapple		
Parsley	Tangerines		
Peas	Tomatoes		
Peppers	Watermelon		
Pumpkins			
Sea vegetables			
Spinach			
Sprouts			
Wheatgrass			

Researchers at Norwich Medical School, University of East Anglia in the United Kingdom, investigated the association between muscle mass and a high dietary intake of alkaline foods. The study published in 2013 in *Osteoporosis International* found that fat-free mass (muscle) was positively associated with a more alkaline diet in healthy women—independent of age, physical activity, and protein intake. The researchers concluded that protein isn't the only player in maintaining muscle mass. Fruits and vegetables rich in potassium and magnesium were also relevant for maintaining muscle mass.

When to Eat

Continue the three-meals-a-day, two-snacks-a-day timing outlined in the liver cleanse. Because your cortisol levels naturally rise at about 8 a.m., you may not feel hungry in the morning, but make sure you eat a protein breakfast before 10 a.m. You have fasted overnight and need to recharge your batteries with good-quality fuel.

An early lunch (before 1:30 p.m.) is better than a late lunch. The midafternoon snack should be between 2 p.m. and 3 p.m. Ideally, you should have dinner before 6:30 p.m. If you find this impossible to do, eat part of your dinner at this time while you're preparing dinner (or on your way home). How? I pack the vegetable portion of my dinner in a sandwich bag to eat in the car on the way back from working at my clinic.

If you don't feel hungry at the time you're supposed to eat, just nibble a few bites of nutrient-dense foods. This will spoon-feed your adrenals and keep your metabolism revved up and burning calories.

Nutrition Schedule

This is what each day on the adrenal healing program looks like.

1. **Morning**

Drink detox tea. Green tea or herbal tea can be substituted, if necessary. If you crave salt, stir ¼ or ½ teaspoon of sea salt in an eight-ounce glass of water as soon as you get up (and before enjoying your tea). A bout of nausea after drinking the salt water indicates that your body doesn't need the salt.

My patients with adrenal fatigue share the same experience in the mornings. They feel more tired when they wake up than they did when they went to sleep. They all say that it takes at least an hour and more than one cup of coffee to feel "awake." Most of them benefit if they can sleep, or at least stay in bed, until 9 a.m. But that is often impossible. Even when we can "sleep in," our brains are programmed, from the busy week, to get up. As a result, getting to bed before 11 p.m. is very important to allow the rest and recuperation time we need. Remember, we are tired not because we're lazy or not pushing hard enough. If you had an injured ankle, you would not go to the gym to work out. You would honor that injury and take care of it. I want you to realize that feeling tired in the morning is often a sign of adrenal fatigue. Treat yourself kindly, gently, and with understanding. The great news is that your adrenals *will* heal, and mornings will soon be a time to anticipate, instead of dread.

2. Breakfast

Eat protein, micronutrients, and good fats. Sauté eggs in olive or grapeseed oil. Cottage cheese with fruit is another option, but do not eat too much dairy in the last half of the thirty-day program if you want to lose weight. Or enjoy a protein smoothie with fresh or frozen berries or other fruit you have hanging around, plus organic, unsweetened almond, coconut, cashew, hemp, or rice milk. Add a scoop of protein mix free from heavy-metal contamination. There are many good options available in health-food stores or online. And take the mixture with you in your coffee cup and have protein in your coffee. I do not recommend soy milk unless it's labeled "nongenetically modified" or "organic." Or mix nonfat Greek yogurt in the smoothie to add protein and creaminess (if you're not lactose-intolerant).

Tea is better than coffee for your adrenals in the morning, and green tea has a little caffeine. Remember, you're on the plan for only fifteen days. I will discuss bringing coffee back into your life and how to maintain your renewed energy in Chapter 10. No sugar or other sweeteners are allowed, but you can use Stevia (preferably) or honey.

3. Midmorning Snack Around 10:30 A.M.

Eat a few bites of protein, good fat, and natural sugar (such as apple slices and almond butter), or veggies (like carrots or cut-up celery) and hummus.

4. Lunch, Ideally Between Noon and 1:30 P.M.

Choose protein (such as chicken) sautéed with lots of brightly colored veggies like kale, bell peppers, tomatoes, or a bean salad. Beans are full of protein. If you want a sandwich, make it whole-grain bread, and open-faced with only one slice. No bagels or whole wheat bread, both of which turn into sugar. Add sprouts, avocado, and veggies to the protein on your sandwich to make it filling and nutrient-dense.

Sprouts are a living food, and have amazing health-promoting qualities. Experts estimate that sprouts have as much as one hundred times more enzymes (which are types of proteins that act like catalysts for all your body's functions) than fruits and vegetables. Sprouts are also full of oxygen and are very alkaline. See pages 236–239 for an easy way to always have fresh sprouts at home.

5. Midafternoon Snack Before 3 P.M.

This snack, which is similar to the midmorning snack, must be timed before the 3 p.m. crash. You're supposed to have a small natural drop in cortisol production around 3 p.m., but you're not supposed to crash. The snack provides an energy boost.

6. Dinner by 6:30 P.M. if Possible

An early dinner is better for your digestion, aids sleep, and is congenial to your circadian rhythm. Eat protein and vegetables from the list, along with salad. Fruit can be your dessert.

7. Evening Snack Between 8 P.M. and 9:30 P.M. (Optional)

If you have sleep problems, nibble a small protein snack like a few spoonfuls of Greek yogurt. If you feel truly hungry, your body is signaling that your blood sugar is low and you need to eat something. However, do not have a snack if you go to bed at 10 p.m. and have no trouble falling asleep. Ask yourself, "Am I really hungry?" Most of what we think of as hunger is actually a craving, or the feeling that the stomach is simply not full.

Supplements

On Days 16–30, take these regardless of how you scored on the adrenal health test. All are available at health-food stores, drugstores, and/or on my website, drtami.com.

Vitamins/Minerals

✧ **B Vitamins**
  a) **B6.** Take 50–100 mg daily.
  b) **Niacin.** Take 25–50 mg daily. Niacin can make some people flush (turn red and feel like the skin is prickly). If this happens, you can buy a non-flushing type, such as niacin hexanol.
  c) **Pantothenic Acid.** Take 1,500 mg per day.
  d) **B Complex.** Take 1,500 mg a day. Because it is a challenge to take all the B vitamins, I recommend taking a B complex that combines multiple B vitamins in one pill.

✧ **Vitamin C.** Start with 500 mg per day and increase to 1,000–2,000 mg per day, every other day. If you experience diarrhea or loose stools, it's a sign that you're taking too much and need to reduce the dose. The dose of vitamin C is different for everyone and depends on how much your body needs and how much you're getting from the foods you eat. You can't get enough by eating oranges. And I don't recommend orange juice or fruit juices, which are actually hard on the adrenals because they bring on a sugar blast—and then you crash.

- ✧ **Vitamin E.** Take 800 units per day of mixed tocopherol. Tocopherol is the technical name for vitamin E.
- ✧ **Calcium.** Take 750 mg per day of calcium citrate or calcium lactate.
- ✧ **Magnesium.** Take 400 grams per day (before bed) of magnesium citrate.
- ✧ **Trace Minerals.** Follow the instructions on the bottle for dosage, as there are many dose strengths available. The minerals important to the adrenals include manganese, selenium, molybdenum, chromium, copper, zinc, and iodine. You can find a mineral supplement that includes all of these.
- ✧ **Fiber.** Mild constipation is often present when you experience adrenal fatigue. Fiber from your green smoothies or citrus pectin will help.

Herbs

- ✧ **Ashwagandha.** Take 500–1,000 mg daily.
- ✧ **Gingerroot.** Take fresh ginger, available at your local grocery store, in tea or add to smoothies or dishes you cook. For tea, take one teaspoon of grated or sliced ginger in a cup of steaming hot water for fifteen minutes. Honey or other natural sweeteners can be added to suit your taste.
- ✧ **Licorice Root.** Start with a small amount and gradually work up to 1/4 teaspoon solid licorice-root extract three times per day. Monitor blood pressure with a home BP device or at your local drugstore if you have blood-pressure problems, as licorice may raise blood pressure in susceptible individuals.

- ✧ **Siberian Ginseng Root.** Take 100–200 mg two to three times a day. Look for ginseng with at least 0.8 percent eleutherosides (the active ingredient). In some people, ginseng can have a stimulatory effect. If that happens, be sure to take your last dose before 3 p.m. Siberian ginseng is not recommended for those with high blood pressure.
- ✧ **DHEA.** Take 5–10 mg daily, but you might need up to 25 mg. The side effect of too much DHEA is acne. If you find that you have a few breakouts, stop for two days and then reduce your dose.

The Easy Way

The list above is for your education, but it is unrealistic (and expensive) to purchase a bottle of each of these items. Fortunately, there are several good adrenal supplements available that have combined many of the items listed. Some even include glandular extracts, which are an added benefit. Extracts are the oldest and most reliable way of helping the adrenals. They were used (and written up in the literature) one hundred years ago. My favorites are Adreno-Mend, from Douglas Laboratories, Doctor Wilson's adrenal supplements. To learn more and see the adrenal boost I created, check my website, drtami.com, under supplements.

Lifestyle

Stress undermines hormone production by the adrenal glands—and your general health. I encourage you to look at aspects of your life that are beneficial and other areas that are negatives for you—anything from smoking to your job, spouse, or friends. Take a sheet of paper, make two columns, and list what occurs to you. Eliminate as many items from your "bad" list as possible. It will make your 30-Day Plan more successful. You may find that you are unable to remove some of the things on your "bad for me" list, such as your boss. In these cases, remember that you only have control over yourself. By actively choosing to be where you are, you give yourself power—and that has been shown to lower stress.

Sleep and Healing Adrenals

Sleep deprivation is rampant in our culture. And, surprisingly, it isn't just how much you sleep but also when you sleep that counts. Unless you get your butt to bed by 10 p.m., there's no chance you can spend enough time in the deep rejuvenative stages of sleep before your body starts raising your cortisol to begin waking up.

In addition, many of us with fatigued adrenals get our second wind around 11 p.m. Fortunately, there's a supplement called Cortisol Manager (Integrative Therapeutics) that is magical for sleep and handling stress. It's a group of herbs that work together in the form of an adaptogen, which boosts when it needs to boost and calms when it needs to calm. Basically, anybody can try Cortisol Manager, which is available online. If it improves your sleep, keep taking it. Take one capsule at night (and go up to two, if necessary) half an hour to a few minutes before you go to bed. There are no side effects. Patients tell me, "I'm so grateful I lost twelve pounds, and I no longer have hot flashes. But that Cortisol Manager is the best thing you've ever recommended." Sleep and weight are tied together. When you sleep better, you lose more weight. Sleep deprivation has been directly correlated with weight gain in countless studies. The size of your brain literally shrinks if you get less than seven hours of sleep a night. Sleep is one of the best anti-aging activities you can do.

Patients say, "Oh, I don't need seven hours. I can get by on six (or four)." And I say the goal is not to give your body what you can get by on. If you bought a million-dollar racehorse, would you give it just enough nourishment to get by on? Or would you buy the best feed available? If you owned a Lamborghini, would you fill the tank with the lowest grade of gas? I don't have a Lamborghini, but if I did I would treat it with more respect.

Here are some other tips for a great night's sleep:

1. Be sure to get physical exercise during the day. Do about thirty minutes of light exercise, like walking, daily.
2. Try to breathe fresh air every day, even if it's raining.
3. Do not watch TV, use your iPad, phone, or anything with a backlight thirty to sixty minutes before going to bed.
4. Sleep in a completely dark room.
5. Try melatonin if you have trouble falling asleep. See page 209 in Chapter 10 to learn how to determine your melatonin dose.

Breathe, Meditate, and Try Tai Chi

When your stress response never rests, your adrenals (those poor little walnut-size glands) say, "Seriously?!"—and partially shut down. Production of all your hormones drops drastically.

But you can change that scenario. On Day 16, start Take Five belly-breathing exercises five times a day. I know. You're saying, "How am I going to find time to do this five times a day?" Don't worry. I have an easy plan for you. Take one to three belly breaths when you wake up in the morning and when you're in your bed before falling asleep. Then breathe before you eat a meal. You can really go for it, and also do breathing before your midmorning and midafternoon snacks.

Take Five exercises lower your heart rate and blood pressure, and literally erase the stress and inflammation from the day. This exercise can also prevent or help manage diabetes, because the adrenal glands play an important role in balancing sugars.

In addition to helping to heal the adrenals, breathing exercises give your liver a break and increase digestive resistance to infection, help with rest and recuperation, and aid in circulation to the skin.

Meditation

The benefits of meditation go far beyond the time spent on the activity. "When you learn meditation, you start de-stressing. Your awareness increases, and your perception of reality changes. You become more carefree," Pedram Shojai, a doctor of oriental medicine, told me. Dr. Shojai lectures throughout the world, teaching people how to improve their lives. He compares meditation to making deposits of carefree feelings and happiness into the bank called "your life."

He explains stress and meditation as "energy economics." He believes we "live our lives on credit," because we continually borrow energy from tomorrow to make up for health and vitality we do not have today. There really is no way to "make up" lost sleep on the weekend, no way to eat a better meal to make up for skipping breakfast, and no way to undo the damage from inflammation that occurs when living a stressful life. As credit accrues from this borrowing, it leads to disease and decline. We eventually experience energy bankruptcy. Our vitality account is empty. This is what happens in adrenal fatigue.

Meditate once a day (to start) for ten minutes. If your score on the adrenal health self-test indicates a serious adrenal-fatigue problem, you will benefit from meditating twice a day for ten minutes each time. Other ways to meditate if you are very busy include listening to guided meditation or listening to Holosync, which I discuss in Chapter 4.

Meditation is one of the most powerful things you can do for your brain, your body, and your health.

Tai Chi and Qigong

Tai chi is a low-impact, slow-motion exercise often described as "meditation in motion." It originated as a martial art in China, and growing evidence shows its value in treating or preventing many health problems. It's the perfect form of exercise for any level of fitness. Deep breathing is built into the movements, as is attention focus. The movements are circular and never forced; the muscles are relaxed, not tensed; and the extensions are gentle, not strained.

A 2006 study published in *Alternative Therapies in Health and Medicine* reported on the benefits of tai chi. Stanford University researchers studied thirty-nine men and women, average age sixty-six, with below-average fitness and at least one cardiovascular risk factor. After taking thirty-six tai chi classes in twelve weeks, they showed improvement in both lower-body strength (measured by the number of times they could rise from a chair in thirty seconds) and upper-body strength (measured by their ability to do arm curls).

In a Japanese study using the same strength measures, 113 older adults were assigned twelve weeks of different exercise programs, including tai chi, brisk walking, and resistance training. Those who did tai chi improved more than 30 percent in lower-body strength and 25 percent in arm strength—almost as much as those who participated in resistance training and more than those assigned to do brisk walking.

Tai chi decreases stress and anxiety, increases energy and stamina, improves quality of sleep, and lowers blood pressure and cholesterol. You can learn tai chi from a video, or take a class at a community or fitness center or health club.

Because meditation, breathing, tai chi, and qigong trigger the relaxation response, they are powerful ways of relieving stress, which can partially shut down the adrenals, and also reduce cortisol levels. Note that qigong and tai chi are often easier for our action-oriented brains, and they serve as "moving" meditation. Another benefit is that these exercises require us to use our large muscles, as they include deep knee bends and flowing low-to-the-ground movements. The movements decrease fat and increase large-muscle mass. Building muscle through movement and exercise has been shown in studies to increase testosterone levels.

The Beginning of Adrenal Health

Your adrenal glands must be healthy in order to manufacture the levels of testosterone and other hormones you need. My patients get results in as little time as a few weeks. However, moderate to severe adrenal fatigue may take anywhere from six months to two years to resolve. In such cases, it is beneficial to incorporate many of the adrenal healing and boosting suggestions in your routine after you complete the 30-Day Plan. But this is a good start. You don't have to sit by helplessly feeling foggy, fatigued, and fat. You can restore your adrenals to optimal health.

CHAPTER 9

Part III: Resetting Hormones

(Days 16–30: Concurrently with Adrenal Repair)

✧ Take specific herbs, vitamins/minerals, and other supplements, depending on the results of your hormone self-tests.

✧ Increase lean protein and eliminate sugar to boost testosterone.

✧ Eat estrogen-friendly and progesterone-friendly foods if indicated, and avoid foods that inhibit these hormones.

✧ Exercise moderately.

Remember the old children's story "The Three Bears"? Goldilocks walked into a house in the woods and found three bowls of porridge. The first bowl was much too hot. The second bowl was much too cold. But the third bowl was just right. I tell my patients that balancing your hormones is like finding that third bowl. If your level of testosterone (or any other essential hormone) is too low, you want to raise it. If the level is too high, you need to reduce it. The goal is a level that's "just right" for you. Only when you reach that point can your hormones work in harmony to maximize your ability to look, feel, and function at the top of your game.

Now that you've detoxed your liver, you're ready to begin the "balancing act" on Days 16–30—at the same time, you are starting the adrenal healing segment. You do both sections simultaneously, because the adrenals need to be at their best to produce the hormones you need. I want you to boost and balance each hormone, because each has unique properties and functions—and its own requirements for optimal performance. I will review testosterone, estrogen, and progesterone and put each into perspective. Although all hormones decline as we age, they rarely decline in a balanced fashion. You may need more help with one hormone than with another.

Everyone takes the same supplements for the liver cleanse, but not everyone will take the same supplements to boost hormones. Almost every woman over forty needs to boost her testosterone. Only in rare circumstances do women have high testosterone as they age, and it is normally associated with medical conditions such as polycystic ovary syndrome (PCOS). (See pages 179–180 in this chapter for information on PCOS.) But some women need to address testosterone along with estrogen and/or progesterone. I will address low testosterone, as well as the rare cases where testosterone is too high; both high and low estrogen; and low progesterone (high rarely happens). High and low cortisol are covered in Chapter 8, which focuses on healing the adrenals.

Boosting and Balancing Testosterone

What's all the hubbub about testosterone? Testosterone is truly your secret weapon. It increases your energy, boosts your brain, improves your moods, treats depression, helps you lose weight, and revs up your sex life. Boosting your *active* testosterone levels on the 30-Day Plan will rock your life.

Here's a punch list of testosterone's other amazing properties:

1. Testosterone helps balance, optimize, and counter the excess of many of our hormones and body functions. For example, testosterone remodels bone. One kind of estrogen builds bone, but old, crappy bone has to be removed and the new, healthy bone put in. That's what remodeling does. If you just have old bone and new bone, you may not wind up with stronger bone. It's like a callus. It's not good tissue; there's just more of it.

2. Testosterone helps cortisol balance sugar spikes.

3. Testosterone helps you look sleek and fabulous, so your body doesn't produce too much fat and turn testosterone into estrogen.

4. Testosterone helps prevent cancer, especially in women who have had a hysterectomy and take estrogen and progesterone.

5. Testosterone is the key ingredient in energy, vitality, and battling fatigue.

Testosterone is your unsung hero. It quietly makes everything better, but you don't miss the benefits until it's gone. Testosterone is necessary to help other hormones work together.

Supplementation for Testosterone

Before you begin, I'm going to ask you to refer back to the testosterone self-test you took on page 49. A score greater than 4 indicates that you have low testosterone. However, if you are over the age of forty, even if you score 4 or below, I want you to stimulate your testosterone production and/or make more of the testosterone you've got available to your body unless you have PCOS. Why? Because even if you don't have obvious symptoms of deficiency yet, you do have deficiency at the cellular level—which affects your organs as it worsens. It's only a matter of time before symptoms show up. I don't want you to wait that long. Make improvements now, starting with supplementation.

Supplements
The following are the herbs, vitamins, and minerals that have been studied and shown to increase testosterone:

✧ **Ashwagandha.** Take 500–1,000 mg daily. But if you're already taking this herb for adrenal healing, that is sufficient, and there's no need to add more.

- ✧ **Maca.** Take 1,000–2,000 mg daily.
- ✧ **Tribulus.** Take 200–400 mg daily.
- ✧ **Vitamin B Complex (B1, B6, B12).** If you're already taking B complex for the adrenal healing part of the 30-Day Plan, you can use that, but be sure to check that it contains B1, B6, and B12. B vitamins help the adrenals but are an additional special help in boosting testosterone.
- ✧ **DHEA.** Take 5–25 mg daily.
- ✧ **Zinc.** Take 30 mg, balanced with 2 mg of copper, two or three times a day. Zinc inhibits the conversion of testosterone into estrogen.
- ✧ **Vitamin C.** Take 750–2,000 mg daily.
- ✧ **Vitamin D.** Take 2,000 IU daily, which seems to be safe for subjects in studies. However, I do have patients who need 10,000 IU or more daily. The best way to determine dosage is to ask your physician to order a vitamin D 25-OH test. You want your level to be in the optimal range of 50–100 mg/ml.
- ✧ **Chrysin.** This herb prevents testosterone from being converted into estrogen. Chrysin does the job by inhibiting the enzyme aromatase. Take 250 mg of oral chrysin twice a day (or 50 mg/g topical chrysin once a day). Some women can use 5–10 mg of topical progesterone to block the conversion of testosterone to estrogen.

The Shortcut

There are supplement companies that have taken many of the above ingredients and put them together, making it much simpler to get all the benefits you need. For example, I created my own proprietary blend in one packet, which can be found on my website, drtami.com. I strive to make things easier. Other options are:

TestoGain (Douglas Laboratories). Taken by mouth, this supplement contains most of the herbs needed to boost testosterone. It is available online and at your physician's office. Take two capsules a day with food for two weeks.

Or

Testo-Care (Life-Flo). This topical cream is available both online and over the counter. It also combines herbs and other ingredients to boost your own production of testosterone.

Plus

Multivitamin. Take one daily, in addition to either TestoGain or Testo-Care, to provide the vitamins and minerals you need. My favorites are Nutreince (Calton Nutrition) and Ultra Preventive (Douglas Laboratories).

Nutrition

The nutrient-dense foods you're eating to heal your adrenals will help create more testosterone in your body. However, testosterone-friendly nutrition is as much about what *not* to eat as about food recommendations. For example, you need to eliminate sugar in order to elevate your testosterone levels naturally. Studies show that testosterone drops by up to 25 percent after you eat sugar. We eat lots of sugar in the United States—about 130 pounds a year per person.

Avoid toxins such as alcohol and cigarettes. You can enjoy a glass of wine after the 30-Day Plan is completed. Cut saturated fats, too; these are the fats that are solid at room temperature. Remember, however, that not all saturated fats are created equal, and the healthy ones, like coconut oil, actually help raise testosterone levels.

Increasing your lean protein to 100–200 grams (3½ ounces to 7 ounces) per day will boost testosterone. Protein repairs cells, makes new ones, and increases your muscle mass. Foods high in zinc, such as spinach and pumpkin seeds, have been shown to be especially testosterone-friendly. The food highest in zinc is oysters.

But remember, we are boosting adrenal function at the same time we are increasing testosterone—and oysters are not on our adrenal nutrition list.

Lifestyle

The weight you will lose during the liver cleanse and the adrenal healing will automatically help you boost your testosterone level. Fat has aromatase activity, which converts testosterone into estrogen. You gain active testosterone just by losing fat.

Moderate exercise also boosts testosterone. Choose an activity you enjoy, because that will increase the chances you'll do it. For example, I danced professionally in a ballet company before I went to medical school, and I had a few injuries during that time. As a result, it's painful for me to run or do yoga or some other popular activities. My go-to exercise is walking. Walking daily for thirty minutes (briskly, as if you were late for an appointment) is an amazing way to stay fit. Give weight to your honest preferences. If everyone you know is in an aerobics or a Pilates class but these are not for you—listen!

The Stress Component

If you want to boost your testosterone, don't forget to reduce stress. Testosterone is produced in your adrenal glands. When these glands are busy, they don't have time to make it. When you're chronically stressed, even mildly, your body has a slow but constant production of cortisol, and cortisol is catabolic, which means it breaks down tissue. Testosterone is anabolic, building bone, muscle, and other tissue. So they work in opposition.

Stress can be broken down into three components: stress, lack of stress, and turning on the relaxation response. Just because you're not feeling stress doesn't mean you're turning on the relaxation response and switching on production of hormones. You're just stopping the assault, which has nothing to do with healing.

Too Much of a Good Thing: PCOS and Infertility

Excess testosterone is found in a medical condition called polycystic ovary syndrome (PCOS), which affects an estimated seven million women and adolescent girls in the United States, 50 percent of them undiagnosed, according to the nonprofit PCOS Foundation. PCOS is essentially too much androgen (testosterone) and not enough progesterone. This results in a bunch of cysts in the ovaries and hormone imbalances. Consequently, women with PCOS have a very difficult time getting pregnant and maintaining pregnancy.

PCOS tops the list of female endocrine disorders. It's a big concern, because it may increase not only the risk of infertility but also the risk of diabetes, high cholesterol, and a host of other problems. Women with PCOS have a four to seven times higher risk of heart attack as well.

The medical community does not currently have a well-defined diagnostic criteria for PCOS, which means that diagnosis might be difficult if you have this hormonal disorder. Symptoms may include acne, excess hair on the face—and even from the belly button to the pubic area—and crazy periods. The latter may go on and on, or you may have fewer than eight periods a year. But symptoms can vary from one woman to another, depending on ethnicity and other factors.

PCOS is suspected in women with acne, infertility, irregular periods, obesity, and insulin resistance. The cause of the condition is unknown, and there is no cure, although PCOS can be medically managed. Early diagnosis is essential. There is a supplement called TestoQuench that helps lower testosterone levels naturally. Many women feel alone when they have PCOS. An amazing organization for education and support is www.pcosdiva.com, founded by my friend and colleague Amy Medling.

If you suspect that you may have PCOS, but find your testosterone levels are low when measured, it may be because your testosterone is getting converted to DHT. After you have confirmed (with a test) that this is happening, there are specific ways to stop or decrease the activity of the enzyme that converts testosterone to DHT.

Estrogen

Although estrogen is the hormone everyone talks about—and is very important—it is not "the queen bee hormone" most people assume it is. Estrogen drops dramatically in middle age. Women are aware of the decline (along with the drop in progesterone) when their periods become irregular, stop, or symptoms like hot flashes, night sweats, and bladder leakage begin to appear.

Start by looking at your score on the estrogen self-test on page 21. If your score is 5 or more, you have an estrogen deficiency. If your score is less than 5, you may benefit from over-the-counter estriol cream, the weak estrogen, which will reduce hot flashes, vaginal dryness, and take the edge off your feelings of discomfort. Remember, there are three main types of estrogen: estradiol, estrone, and estriol. If you do not have a menstrual cycle, apply topical estriol on Days 1–25 of the calendar to help with symptoms of low estrogen. If you do menstruate, apply estriol daily and stop when you have your period.

Estriol is twenty times less active than the other estrogens. In fact, it's being investigated as a possible treatment for breast cancer because it fits estrogen receptors just like tamoxifen, preventing other strong estrogens from binding.

Vitamins and Minerals

✧ **Vitamin A.** Take 30,000 IU daily.
✧ **Vitamin E.** Take 400 IU daily.

- ✧ **Boron.** Take 3 mg of this mineral twice a day.
- ✧ **Zinc.** Take 30 mg daily, balanced with 2 mg of copper, twice a day. Zinc taken alone can create copper deficiency.

Herbs

These over-the-counter herbs safely stimulate your body to produce estradiol:

- ✧ **Black Cohosh.** Take 40 mg of a standardized extract twice a day.
- ✧ **Chasteberry.** Take 175 mg solid extract daily.
- ✧ **Dong Quai.** Also known as female ginseng, and used for menstruation problems. Follow the directions on the bottle. Caution: It can interact with blood-thinning medications like warfarin.
- ✧ **Maca.** 1,000–2,000 mg daily.
- ✧ **Red Clover.** This is available in a variety of preparations, including teas, tinctures, tablets, capsules, liquid extracts, and extracts standardized to specific isoflavone contents. It can also be prepared as an ointment for topical (skin) application.
  a) Dried herb (used for tea): 1–2 teaspoons dried flowers or flowering tops steeped in 8 ounces of hot water for 30 minutes; drink 2–3 cups daily.
  b) Powdered herb (available in capsules): 40 mg–160 mg daily, or 28–85 mg of red clover isoflavones.
  c) Tincture (1:5, 30 percent alcohol): 60–100 drops (3–5 mL) three times a day. May be added to hot water as a tea.
  d) Fluid extract (1:1): 1 mL three times per day. May be added to hot water as a tea.

Estrogen Dominance

In some women, we find that the other hormones, such as testosterone and progesterone, have declined faster than estrogen, leaving them "unbalanced" and with a "relative" estrogen dominance. Estrogen dominance can also result from receiving hormone treatment after a hysterectomy. Traditionally, women undergoing hysterectomy have been offered estrogen alone, which creates estrogen dominance. The latter is associated with an increase in cancers, especially uterine cancer. The theory is that estrogen dominance does not matter after a hysterectomy because these women no longer have a uterus. But what about the estrogen, progesterone, and testosterone balance in other parts of the body, such as the breasts, the bones, and the brain? Hormones are meant to work together. Replacing only one creates imbalances and does not mimic Mother Nature.

Nutrition

Increase Your Intake of Estrogen-Friendly Foods

✧ Legumes
✧ Soybeans
✧ Bran
✧ Estrogen-friendly fruits and vegetables

Legumes, lentils, and beans are beneficial for estrogen. Soybeans are especially good, because they contain isoflavonoids, a type of phytoestrogen ("phyto" meaning plant-based). Soybeans not only boost estrogen; they have some estrogenic activity and behave like estrogen.

Certain foods contain lignans, which are a type of plant estrogen and a fat-soluble antioxidant. Lignans are found in high concentrations in flaxseeds and sesame seeds, and in smaller amounts in fruits and vegetables like kale and broccoli, apricots, cabbage, Brussels sprouts (and also dark rye bread).

Postmenopausal women who consume diets rich in lignans have a lower risk of breast cancer. Twenty-one studies were reviewed in what is called a meta-analysis. Findings were published in the *American Journal of Clinical Nutrition* in 2010. The conclusion was that higher lignan exposure may be associated with a reduced breast cancer risk in postmenopausal women. Other studies have shown that diets high in lignans also reduce the risk of ovarian cancer and endometrial cancer.

Peas and pinto and lima beans contain coumestan, which is another type of phytoestrogen.

Try to incorporate more vitamin C, carotene, and B-complex-rich foods into your diet because these vitamins are useful in lifting estrogen levels in women (mostly by helping your adrenals). Foods high in vitamin C include kiwis, tomatoes, oranges, cantaloupes, peaches, bananas, artichokes, asparagus, carrots, cauliflower, corn, and lima beans.

Foods rich in carotene include peppers, kale, spinach, carrots, beets, dandelion greens, turnip greens, cabbage, pumpkins, chard, collards, basil, and squash. These are awesome ingredients to toss into your smoothie or into a Crock-Pot to make a yummy soup ready for when you come home from work.

Foods rich in B complex include beets, tuna, oats, turkey, bananas, Brazil nuts, avocados, and legumes.

Eating cruciferous vegetables, such as broccoli, cauliflower, and Brussels sprouts, helps your estrogens become protective against cancer. These veggies help prevent estrogen from becoming the 16-hydroxyestrone procarcinogenic form. On the other hand, if you have too little of 16-hydroxyestrone, your bones will be affected. It's always a balancing act.

Avoid Foods that Inhibit Estrogen Production

These include melons, pineapple, berries, figs, grapes, green beans, corn, white rice, and white flour. Eliminating even one of these foods will increase estrogen production.

SYMPTOMS OF ESTROGEN EXCESS

Some people wind up with too much estrogen. Symptoms include:

❖ Breast tenderness

❖ Crying spells and increased emotional sensitivity

❖ Depression

❖ Endometriosis

❖ Heavy periods with clotting

❖ Infertility

❖ Irregular menstrual cycles

❖ Migraine headaches

❖ Ovarian cysts

❖ Panic attacks

❖ Severe menstrual cramps

❖ Uterine fibroids

❖ Water retention, bloating

❖ Weight gain

Remember, our hormones are designed to work together to balance and protect. It's when we're in our forties and beyond, when our hormones are unbalanced, that we see a rise in cancers associated with hormones.

What to Do If You Have Estrogen Excess

1. Optimize progesterone. Progesterone is the "stop" to estrogen's "go." Estrogen makes cells grow; progesterone halts proliferation. Estrogen causes water retention; progesterone is a natural diuretic. Estrogen elevates your mood; progesterone calms and quiets a stressed, worried mind. Progesterone exits the body first and fastest, so you can have a relative excess of estrogen in perimenopause just because progesterone has left the building.

2. Lose fat. Fat makes estrogen levels rise. Even five pounds off can reduce excess estrogen.

3. Remove xenoestrogens. These are the chemicals that act like bad estrogen in our environment. Canned goods, plastics, cosmetics, skin-care products, and the fire retardant on your furniture all contain the chemicals that act like bad estrogen. Look for plastic that is bisphenol A (BPA)-free, and for skin-care items that do not have parabens (a preservative listed at the end of the ingredients on the package). Eat less canned foods. Xenoestrogens love to hang out in your fat and can remain stored there for years. That is why it's so important to do a liver cleanse.

4. Cleanse your liver. The liver is the main way your body rids itself of excess estrogen.

Because estrogen is intimately connected to serotonin, a chemical in your body that works as a neurotransmitter and is associated with feeling happy, it's not surprising that estrogen deficiency or excess can greatly affect your mood. Even the changes in estrogen levels throughout a menstrual cycle can make a difference. Serotonin is also connected with appetite and sleep, which is why you crave chocolate or carbs and feel more short-tempered before your period.

Estrogen and Birth-Control Pills
Birth-control pills are an individual choice. But, if you take them, understand that they are composed of synthetic estrogen, which is estrogen extracted from the urine of a pregnant mare. Our bodies are amazing at recognizing a foreign substance—and estrogen from a horse is foreign. Many reactions to the intrusion can take place, such as breast tenderness, weight gain, irregular bleeding, and headaches (including migraines).

In addition, taking synthetic estrogens by mouth has been shown to increase sex hormone-binding globulin (SHBG), which preferentially holds on to testosterone and estrogen, reducing active hormone levels. Birth-control pills affect testosterone levels right away.

The Question of Soy

Soy is great for estrogen activity, but its health benefits are widely debated. The majority of soy products we see are genetically modified. (Soy became genetically modified in 1996.) And we still do not know the true risk of genetically modified foods. These foods have been banned in many countries, including much of Europe, because their safety remains unproven. However, genetically modified foods are allowed in the United States because there is no proof of harm. We do know that early animal medical studies show that genetic modification of food inhibits fertility. Genetically modified foods are different. If soy milk is certified-organic soy, then you're probably safe. It's your way of knowing that this has been inspected. It's what it says it is, is not genetically modified, and is not contaminated. But look at the package. If there's no certified-organic label, it's great marketing—which guarantees nothing.

I currently advise using natural soy foods like tofu rather than supplements. But you still have to be careful, because sometimes soy is not considered a food product and is not inspected as such. Soy is also often imported from China, where the criteria for contamination and consistency are far below our standards for food safety.

To make your life easier, I have created an online shopping cart for foods and other items, which you can find on my website, drtami.com.

Relative estrogen dominance plus testosterone decline can also make you gain weight. In addition, our fat acts like an organ and produces a hormone that takes the little testosterone you do have and converts it into even more estrogen, which produces more fat. And so the cycle goes on and on. That's one of the reasons we gain weight after forty.

Boosting Progesterone

Progesterone deficiency in young women can give them heavy, painful periods, PMS, and infertility—and also cause miscarriages. After forty, one of the first signs of deficiency is often an inability to sleep through the night or difficulty in "keeping your cool." The latter symptom is often overlooked in professional women with and without children. In my own life, I thought my increased frustration and irritability were due to being the mother of two young children, as well as being a physician with a busy practice. How my life changed when I boosted my own progesterone levels!

Progesterone is really hard to make. It's a prized jewel stolen by the adrenal glands to produce more cortisol. Your adrenals produce cortisol at every perception of stress throughout the day. When the adrenals run out of ingredients to make as much cortisol as our 24/7 lifestyle requires, they kidnap the raw ingredients in progesterone (and testosterone and estrogen, too) to make more cortisol. This increased cortisol subsequently blocks progesterone from its receptors, preventing this amazing hormone from entering our cells to do its work.

Progesterone has many functions on its own, including raising your body temperature and boosting your metabolism. It also plays an important part in regulating estrogen. When progesterone levels decrease faster than estrogen, we become estrogen-dominant. This leaves us at an increased risk for endometrial cancer, breast tenderness, moodiness, and endometriosis.

Check your results on the progesterone self-test on page 25. If your score is 6 or higher, you need to boost your progesterone through supplementation. I took all of these for my own progesterone deficiency:

Vitamins and Minerals

✧ **Vitamin B6.** (This may be included in your B complex.) Take 200–800 mg per day.

✧ **Vitamin C.** Take 750 mg per day. A dose of 750–1,000 mg has been shown in studies to raise progesterone in women.

✧ **Selenium.** Take 200–400 mcg per day, which was shown to boost production of progesterone in an Italian study.

Herbs

✧ **Chasteberry.** Take 500–1,000 mg per day.

✧ **Turmeric.** Thyme and oregano are also useful for progesterone. Use in cooking whenever you can.

Topical progesterone cream is also available over the counter as a supplement in place of or in addition to the above.

Nutrition

Eat Progesterone-Friendly Foods

There are no studies of specific foods to boost progesterone, but it has been found that these foods boost progesterone because they're rich in the vitamins needed to make it: cherries, walnuts, chicken, yams, turmeric, thyme, and oregano.

Eat good fats, such as olive oil and nuts, which provide good dietary cholesterol. Increase your intake of foods rich in B vitamins, such as salmon, broccoli, and red peppers. An optimized thyroid also increases progesterone levels.

Avoid Foods that Decrease Progesterone

Saturated fats decrease progesterone levels, as does overeating. One study found that weight loss increased progesterone levels and led to resumed ovulation in 87 percent of infertile patients. If you eat conventional foods like meat and foods from animal products, such as cheese and dairy, choose organic and grass-fed products to avoid hormone intake that can create a hormone imbalance.

A recent case in my practice involved Dana, a thirty-six-year-old married banker who came to see me about her weight, sleep, and sex life. She had no children and traveled a lot. She gained ten pounds "out of nowhere" and could not sleep through the night. The fun had gone out of her marriage, although she loved her husband deeply. She also reported tender swollen breasts, bloating, and feeling tired around the time of her period.

Dana's self-assessment showed many signs of estrogen dominance and a progesterone deficiency. I gave her a blood test that confirmed both. Dana was not interested in bioidentical hormones, which are the same as your body's own natural hormones and are not synthetic. They are created in compounding pharmacies. She felt that, in her thirties, she should be able to treat this "naturally."

After Dana did a cleanse, we took an honest look at her food intake. She increased fresh vegetables, fruits, and lean protein. She also took progesterone-boosting herbs and vitamins. We removed xenoestrogens by looking at her makeup and skin-care products. Dana lost eight pounds in one month, and felt better than she had in years.

I wasn't surprised. Progesterone plays a crucial role both in balancing estrogen and in your quality of life.

Act Now

You don't have to wait until you have no sex life and osteoporosis, no energy and a fat, soft belly to realize that you need testosterone! We all do. It is the secret way to increase vitality, get better brain function, lose weight, and increase libido. Remember the study showing that testosterone protects against breast cancer? Your body won't make too much if you just encourage production. There isn't a woman over forty who can't benefit.

As you get older you also get estrogen-dominant, with little or no progesterone, so balance is gone. You have a relative excess of estrogen. These hormones all work together, and you want to fine-tune them accordingly.

Add It Up

The 30-Day Plan gives you a whole new start at revitalizing your body systems through cleansing, healing, and rebalancing. If you've completed the 30-Day Plan, you now have:

1. A squeaky-clean liver, primed to work at full capacity to filter all the chemicals and toxins you breathe, eat, and absorb every day.
2. Adrenal glands well on the way to regaining health. Full recovery takes more time if you have severe adrenal fatigue, but healing is in progress.
3. Testosterone, estrogen, and progesterone at levels nature intended at your age—and rebalanced to work in harmony.
4. Loss of eight to ten pounds, weight that has slipped away without dieting.
5. More focus and energy, and have found the "fun" part of life again.

The journey from fine to fabulous is not as hard as one might think!

CHAPTER 10

What's Next?

Good intentions come and go. Enthusiasms fade. Resolutions soar, and then fizzle. The challenge is to use the 30-Day Plan as a launching pad for a new way of life, and continue with it to keep the benefits rolling in on a permanent basis. I can hear you saying now, "I will. I will." But because human nature is what it is, here are some guidelines to help keep you on track—patient-tested strategies that factor in the realities and stresses of life today.

If you've followed the 30-Day Plan (picking and choosing doesn't count), you've lost weight as promised, and look and feel noticeably better than you have in a very long time. The clock never stops ticking, yet women tell me they haven't felt so young and vital since their twenties.

How can you keep that momentum going? First, let's take a look at your priorities. Are you feeling great and looking your best? Do you want to preserve these results? Are you now satisfied with your weight, and do you simply want to maintain it? Do you want to lose more weight or have a firmer body or a better brain or stronger bones? Do you want to feel more energized or more confident or sexier from now on? Do you want continuing, safe relief from hot flashes—or to sleep better? You're likely to have more than one priority, but let's take these goals one at a time.

Eat for the Long Haul

The great news about eating nutrient-dense foods—and eating often—is that it accomplishes more than one goal. You take charge of your hunger and make it manageable. Because you nourish your cells, you boost your brain, strengthen your bones, and banish the 3 p.m. crash. You're more productive because it's as if you have more hours of high-octane energy all day. And, because you are fueling your tank without long periods of "empty time," you don't enter the stress zone where your body must produce cortisol, which turns on you and puts fat on your belly.

Without exception, after my patients complete this program they say they are shocked at how much they eat and how great they feel inside and out.

The rules for nutrient-dense eating presented in Chapter 6 are a template to live by for the rest of your life. They include:

1. Wake up to green tea.
2. If you *love* coffee, have one cup and put protein in it. Some people insist on this one-cup-per-day enjoyment. The protein will buffer the effects of the caffeine on your adrenals, and give you the morning protein you need as well. There are several protein powders on the market for you to try, but many do not dissolve well in hot liquids like coffee. I have one that I created for my husband, who cannot dream of a day without coffee. Now he can start his day with coffee *and* protein. It is available on my website, drtami.com, but you can try any of the ones you already have.
3. Have protein for breakfast. Remember the eggs and protein shakes I told you about.
4. Snack at midmorning. Low-glycemic fruits and nuts, veggies and hummus are great options. Don't fall back on protein bars and processed snacks, even if they are labeled "healthy." Your body needs real food.

5. Have lunch no later than 1:30 p.m.

6. Snack before 3 p.m. Choose among the same snack options as for midmorning, or take a shake break of a green smoothie or a real fruit protein smoothie.

7. Satisfy "before dinner hunger" (if you have it) around 5 p.m. More veggies here with some good fats, like a handful of almonds or an avocado.

8. Eat dinner by 6:30 p.m. If you do not want to lose any more weight, slowly add grains. I recommend using ancient grains, which are full of protein, whenever possible. For example, quinoa pasta tastes delicious and is great for you. Farro (or emmer) is an ancient wheat that sustained the Roman legions. It can be served in place of rice.

If you do eat gluten products, remember that they are a treat. I believe far fewer people are sensitive to gluten than the current buzz would have us believe. The truth is that our bodies have zero requirements for simple carbohydrates such as bread, pasta, and rice. Everything we need to thrive can be found in nuts, beans, legumes, fruit, vegetables, meat, and fish. These foods feed your cells. All the rest feed our satisfaction—so enjoy, but keep it within bounds. Bulgur and buckwheat are other ancient grains. These grains are different from modern grains because they're packed with protein. We survived as a species because we were able to eat these grains, which are nutrient-dense. In contrast, modern grains that we eat today (because we prefer fluffy bread) are no longer full of nutrition. Today's wheat does not resemble the wheat of eighty years ago.

The ancient grains haven't been ruined, because they've been out of fashion. Quinoa is exactly the same as it was two hundred years ago. Ancient grains not only feed your cells; their flavor can be satisfying, and they make you feel full. If you eat white bread, you're hungry an hour later. It spikes your insulin, and then you crash.

If you have trouble sleeping (and only then), eat some yogurt with berries and stevia around 9 p.m. if you want it sweetened.

We have to use our eating time and the room we have in our stomach to eat micronutrients. When you get to the point where you've lost weight, you can include ancient grains in your diet. It's not about deprivation. It's about replacement.

If everybody is having pasta and you want some, have it. But the portion should fit inside your palm, not the size of your plate. That's your serving size for grain. And water is the fluid to drink, not soda or Crystal Light. Ideally, you should drink sixty-four ounces of water a day.

Follow the 90 Percent/10 Percent or 80 Percent/20 Percent Rule

I know that you're not going to stick with a permanent seven-day-a-week nutrition-dense goal. Our society makes that almost impossible, with our fast-paced life and the less-than-best quick-food options available. Which is why I don't ask you to. Instead, I say, "Make 90 percent of what goes into your mouth each day healthy food. Designate the other 10 percent for satisfaction only." Or, if necessary, make it 80 percent/20 percent. The same rule works on a weekly basis if you prefer that. Make 10 percent or 20 percent of what you eat each week foods that you love but don't qualify as "nutritious." I'm talking about foods like chocolate, ice cream, cakes, and steak once in a while. But you've gone too far off track if you try the 90/10 or 80/20 formula by the month. The point is to be flexible and realistic so you can continue to succeed. Sticking with this rule (at least most of the time) ensures that you can stay in control of your weight. You may say, "Okay, I'll eat just fruits and vegetables and protein." But even some fruits, such as watermelon, have a high-glycemic index. In order to lose weight, you want to eat

foods that have a glycemic index of 50 or less most of the time—
the 90-percent part.

Women are so hard on themselves. If you have a piece of cake at
work, you say, "My diet is blown today. I will start again tomorrow."
I say stop, be kinder and more flexible with yourself. If you want to
enjoy a piece of cake that was brought to work (and you aren't trying
to lose more weight), then do so. Try not to eat the entire piece, as
you can probably feel satisfied with a portion and then say, "Good.
That was the satisfaction part of my day. Now I am going to stick
with the 80 percent of nutrient-dense foods, because I deserve to feel
fabulous." And if you want to be a rock star, shoot for 90 percent/10
percent.

Saying Yes Increases Success

After you've completed the 30-Day Plan, you will feel an increase
in energy, and it will be easier to avoid the foods that make you feel
bad. But when you really want a treat, say yes. Yes to a small piece of
chocolate (not the entire bar); yes to one small scoop of ice cream.
When your body says, "I want some more," tell it "Yes—tomorrow."
Yes opens doors and allows you to be patient. "No" feels like hold-
ing your breath or gritting your teeth, and cannot be sustained long-
term. Another satisfying trick I use is to take some frozen apples and
cinnamon and combine them with water for "apple water." Use your
tongue and your taste buds to experience flavor. When people want
to lose weight, they usually create a very bland diet. They fall off it
because they crave flavor.

Get Into the Smoothie/Juicing Habit

I saw a patient recently who had just finished a successful weight-loss
effort with me, and we were talking about maintenance. I said, "You

have to start your day with protein." She assured me, "I do. I have a shake." When I asked what was in her shake, she replied, "Oh, I have a banana and a few strawberries." I said, "That's not enough. You have to pack the shake with micronutrients and protein. One medium banana has less than 2 grams of protein. Add raspberries, blueberries, apples, and a scoop of protein powder to get more of those micronutrients into your body." The average adult woman needs a minimum of about 46 grams of protein a day, much more if she wants to lose weight.

According to Vitamix Corporation, an ongoing online study of blended drinks by ORC International found that we Americans made a total of 3.42 billion smoothies with fruits and vegetables at home from July 2013 to June 2014. That figure is undoubtedly much higher today, as more and more of us buy juicers and blenders. If price is no object, you can buy smoothies and juices that are freshly prepared while you wait. According to *Barron's*, more than 6,200 juice bars or smoothie shops have sprung up in big cities and suburbs. In New York, these bars seem to be on every street corner, and even in upscale gyms. However, you'll pay up to $10–$13 or more for a fresh protein drink or a green smoothie, and you need to be very careful, as the ingredients often have hidden sweeteners. Economically, that's a hardship for most of us. It's not only cheaper but more convenient to do it yourself at home.

I know it's hard to wrap your head around another chore in your busy day. It may take you a while to make the commitment. But I urge you to keep it on your to-do list. When you're in the mood, shop around online and in stores and educate yourself in the types of machines available and the range of prices. You can get a simple version, like the NutriBullet, for less than $100 or spend more than $600 for a model with all the bells and whistles.

Walk into a health-food store and check out the smoothie and juicing ingredients I've suggested, such as protein powder (which is available in small individual packets or large containers) and coconut milk. My patient Patty was shocked at the variety available. It can be confusing at first, so head directly for a store employee and ask for guidance. Many supermarkets today also carry certain ingredients. It's not unusual to find three different kinds of coconut water in a grocery store. Fare for "health-food nuts" has definitely gone mainstream. A friend of mine even found kale salad on a Caribbean cruise.

As for chilled bottled smoothies and juices on sale in supermarkets and other stores, until recently most of these products were pasteurized and designed to be able to sit on the shelf for a long time to make them profitable. However, the pasteurization process that kills harmful bacteria (a good thing) also kills many of the living enzymes and nutrients (a bad thing). But since I started writing this book numerous companies have begun making unpasteurized juice—even Starbucks. It's everywhere now. Preferably, the juice should be cold-pressed unpasteurized.

I can honestly tell you that creating a smoothie habit is not a hugely time-consuming thing. I put all the ingredients into my NutriBullet at night, refrigerate, and simply blend it in the morning and drink while I'm preparing my kids' lunches for school and getting ready to go to my clinic to see patients.

Patty got into the routine in stages. She shopped around for an inexpensive machine for months before buying one on sale. She'd never tasted dandelion greens before, but she bought and tried them for her first homemade smoothie (along with cucumber and apple)—and then moved on to Swiss chard, another "mystery vegetable" to her. Now she's exploring chia seeds. "It's a whole new world," she told me.

Check What's in Your Refrigerator

You're not going to change your eating habits unless you shop differently and keep healthy foods on hand. Take inventory of your refrigerator and your pantry shelves. Many single women who live alone have shelves full of prepared and processed foods. The philosophy is: "It's only me." You need to change that attitude if you want to change your life. Protein bars aren't going to do it. For the 30-Day Plan, you stocked up on kale, spinach, peppers, onions, tomatoes, apples, pears, blueberries, and other nutrient-dense foods. Don't stop now and go back to old ways.

Use Food-Evaluation Tools

Get into the habit of evaluating what you eat. Use your search engine to check the protein content of fruits and vegetables when making juices and smoothies. Do the same to determine the glycemic-index rating for various foods. (Every food has a glycemic-index rank.) Check whether particular foods are alkaline or acidic as well. And be sure to have at least one green drink a day. Your cells will thank you.

Preserve Your Nutrients Tip

We have a tendency in this country to eat leftovers. We heat and reheat, which reduces the nutrient density of foods. To preserve the nutrition, try my leftover makeover ideas for a unique take on recipes: There is no reheating involved in these.

I. TOMORROW'S CHICKEN

Serve chicken marsala (the recipe can be found at drtami.com) with two brightly colored vegetables, salad, and farro cooked in organic chicken broth. The next day, dice up the leftover chicken, add chopped celery and mayo, a few dried cranberries, and make chicken salad with a side of quinoa and a piece of fruit or a serving of sorbet for dessert. If you're trying to lose weight, choose the fruit, not the sorbet.

2. ROCCO'S LASAGNA

Meat Sauce:

I double the recipe of the meat sauce, as it freezes very well and is amazing on so many things.

- 2 onions, quartered, and ½ cup fresh basil leaves (If you do not have fresh basil, use 1 heaping tablespoon of prepared pesto and 1 tablespoon of Italian seasoning.)
- 2 tablespoons olive oil
- 1 pound organic ground beef or turkey
- 2 garlic cloves minced, or ½ to 1 teaspoon of already minced garlic
- 6 fresh tomatoes, seeded and chopped (about 4 cups), or organic canned tomatoes
- 2 cups crushed tomatoes (canned or fresh)
- 1 cup dry red wine
- 1 cup chicken stock
- ¼ cup tomato paste
- ½ teaspoon freshly ground black pepper
- Salt to taste
- Pinch of nutmeg
- 5 bay leaves

In a food processor, chop the onions and the basil together and set aside. (No need if you are using prepared pesto.)

In a large pot, heat the oil over high heat and brown the beef, breaking it up with a spoon. Add the onion mixture and the garlic; cook, stirring, for about 3 minutes.

Stir in the chopped tomatoes, crushed tomatoes, wine, stock, tomato paste, salt, pepper, nutmeg, and bay leaves.

Bring to a boil; reduce the heat and simmer, stirring occasionally for about 30 minutes or until thickened.

Discard the bay leaves.

Set aside the meat sauce for layering lasagna and for a leftover makeover.

Béchamel Sauce (white sauce) for lasagna:

Makes 2½ cups

- 4 tablespoons (½ stick) butter
- 1/3 cup potato flour
- 1½ cups milk
- 2 egg yolks
- 1½ cups shredded Parmesan and/or Asiago cheese
- Freshly ground black pepper

In a saucepan, melt the butter over medium heat. Stir in the flour; cook, stirring, for 1 minute. Gradually whisk in the milk. Cook, stirring constantly, for 3 minutes or until thickened.

Remove from the heat. In a bowl, whisk the egg yolks to loosen; whisk a small amount of the milk mixture into the egg yolks. Whisk back into the saucepan and return to medium-low heat.

Cook, stirring, for about 2 minutes or until pale and thickened. Remove from the heat and stir in the cheese until melted. Season to taste with pepper.

Cover and keep warm, or warm slightly before assembling the lasagna.

Assembly: First Layer
Butter the bottom of a lasagna baking dish.

Cover the bottom of the dish with a layer of meat sauce.

Cover the meat sauce with white sauce, mixing it together in the baking dish.

Place a layer of cooked quinoa lasagna noodles on top (following package instructions).

Second Layer

Meat sauce

White sauce

Cheese (Parmesan/Asiago mixed cheese)

Noodles

Repeat the second layer instructions for layer three.

You might have room for a fourth layer, but it's not necessary if your pan is shallow.

Cover the top with cheese.

Preheat the oven to 400°F. Bake, covered, for 30 minutes. Remove the cover, reduce the heat to 350°F, and bake for an additional 30 minutes. Remove from the oven and allow 30 minutes for the lasagna to set before serving.

Note: I like to serve the lasagna with a cucumber and carrot salad. Grate cucumbers and carrots, and toss with lemon, honey, and extra virgin olive oil to taste.

3. SPAGHETTI HEAVEN

Spaghetti squash gets its name from the fact that the inside, when cooked, pulls out in long strands like spaghetti. It contains a high amount of vitamin C, A, B6, and other vitamins, minerals, and fiber, making it almost a superfood.

Cook the spaghetti squash by cutting it lengthwise, scraping out the seeds, and baking for 30 to 40 minutes at 375°F.

Using a fork, scrape out the strands of spaghetti squash. Pour the meat sauce left over from the lasagna on the top for an amazing new and healthy leftover makeover.

4. POLLO ALLA CACCIATORE (HUNTER-STYLE CHICKEN)

- 4 tablespoons butter
- 2 tablespoons olive oil
- 1 onion, chopped
- 1 garlic clove, chopped, or ¼ to ½ teaspoon garlic powder
- 4 chicken breasts
- 1 pound crushed tomatoes (can be canned, but look for ones that do not have BPA)
- ½ pound fresh porcini mushrooms, or 4 ounces dried, cut into pieces
- Salt and black pepper to taste
- 4 tablespoons dry white wine

Heat the butter with the oil. Add the onion and garlic, and cook for a few minutes until soft. Add the chicken and brown on all sides. Add the tomatoes and the mushrooms, season to taste, then pour in the wine. Cover and cook slowly over medium heat or in a moderately warm oven (325°F) for about 1 hour.

Leftover Makeover
Put any leftover chicken and tomato into a food processor and mix. Use this mixture to make lettuce wraps with shredded cabbage, avocado, and bell peppers.

These dishes take no more time than reheating, and give you and your family the full benefits of delicious nourishment.

Alcohol, Processed Foods, and Sugar—Oh, My!

Limit alcohol to no more than two drinks in a day (one is even better, and none is the best). We've all heard that red wine, in particular, is good for you, due to the resveratrol it contains. Remember that in order for you to get enough resveratrol from wine to benefit your health and your heart, you would need to drink an excessive amount.

Alcohol is not good for you. You should put it in the chocolate or bread category, meaning that it is something you eat for the pleasure it gives you, not because it has nutritional value. I want to encourage you to make these choices count. If you are eating or drinking a treat, be fully present in the experience. So many of us pop things into our mouths without even realizing we've done it.

Avoid processed foods, which stress your liver. Processed foods are acidic, and most of them easily turn into sugar. You can raise your testosterone levels just by eliminating processed foods and sugar. (Remember, sugar lowers your testosterone levels.) At the very least, reduce your consumption with the 90/10 or 80/20 rule. The interesting thing is that many women find the fewer processed and sugary foods they eat, the less they crave them. It's as if the body adjusts. What you want changes—or how much you want changes. This is because processed foods literally desensitize our taste buds, and we no longer enjoy the taste of real food. When we start eating real food most of the time, suddenly a fresh tomato is a mouthwatering experience because our taste buds can function again!

Dine on wholesome foods in a wholesome way—slowly, with intention, and sitting down. Too many of us stand up while we eat, or grab something on the run, which just adds stress to our lives. My family has a dinnertime tradition. We all take turns telling one another what we are grateful for and describing our favorite part of the day. In studies, gratitude has been shown to have a very positive effect on health and mood, and it slows down the meal to an enjoyable pace.

I was recently told a story by one of my patients. She had changed her relationship with food and was following my guidelines on what to eat and when. She told me that the information I gave her was not new. Her father, one of the first "food inventors," had told her these things a long time ago. He created Miracle Whip and other "food products." When he had a heart attack, he told her he was not surprised, as he felt that it was all the chemicals and unnatural substances lining his arteries that caused it. He urged her to eat differently.

Make the way you eat and enjoy your food matter. If you do, you'll realize that your work is even more successful, because each thing you do is more intentional.

Eating Healthy in Restaurants and While Traveling

My single most powerful piece of advice is: "Order off the menu." When you do, you get fresher food and food that doesn't include added sugar, fat, and salt. Instead of dining on chicken that's been prepared and marinated in saline since 4 a.m., customize your meal. Say, "May I please have roast chicken on a mound of spinach with balsamic vinegar and olive oil, plus any vegetables you have. I don't like onions." Women have a tendency not to want to be a bother. But men have no trouble at all asking for what they want. These days, restaurants are poised to respond to alternative requests, because there are so many food allergies and customers with gluten sensitivity.

One patient told me that she felt embarrassed when she went out with coworkers and didn't want to say, "I can't have this and I can't have that." I told her to call the restaurant the day before to place her order. An advertising executive shared that tip with me. She said, "If you go to a particular restaurant twice a month, they'll be happy to see you. They know you're the one who calls ahead. You're a good customer, and they want you to be happy. They're in the customer-service business." It won't work in a burger joint unless you're going to one that is particularly service-oriented. But try it in other restaurants. It even works at restaurants that you're trying for the first time.

When you're out and about, choose a salad you (or the restaurant) can make fresh, with protein and dressing on the side. If you order a sandwich, get it made fresh, and never buy an already wrapped sandwich. You just don't know when it was made. Remove one of the pieces of bread and eat the sandwich open-faced. You can choose to add butter or mayonnaise if you wish, but avocado is the best alternative. Soups are great options, as long as they aren't creamed.

As for airports and planes, God's travel food is a hard-boiled egg. It's an amazing snack. We now know that eggs are not the high-cholesterol villains they were previously thought to be. The yoke and the white together are a complete protein, an advantage that far outweighs any cholesterol concerns. And don't be fooled by cheese. There's a little bit of protein in it, but you're much better off with a container of hummus and a bag of cut-up veggies. We all have purses. We have no excuses for not throwing some almonds or a small apple into a plastic bag.

Or choose breakfast items in airports even though it's 11 a.m. or 1 p.m. Get the oatmeal, the low-cal egg sandwich, plus plain yogurt and a piece of fruit. Make breakfast your meal to tide you over. You can also bring your own protein-shake powder and mix it with coconut water or milk that's available at airports. Most such products taste terrible when mixed with water, but there are several on the market that taste great, including my own proprietary protein. See drtami.com. We all know when we're going to be on an airplane. Plan ahead and take along a snack. Bring fruit on board if you have food allergies. Drink lots of water. Salads are a good option, too, and this is one time you can have a protein bar.

At times, I may speak at three different conferences in a three-week period. Although you can usually get fruit at conferences, the food choices at airports are terrible. All you see is bagels and pastries. Protein powder takes the edge off hunger, which is due to low blood sugar. You can also find individual foil packs of almond butter, walnut butter, and pecan butter at Trader Joe's or Whole Foods. They're called nut butters. You wouldn't pack for a trip without taking your toothbrush and toothpaste, and you have to think of taking care of your cells.

Preparation Is Paramount

No one plans to fail; they just fail to plan. This is as true for nutrition as for life in general. This tip works for me: When I buy groceries, before I put them in the refrigerator I take ziplock plastic bags and fill them right then and there with cherry tomatoes, snap peas, and cut-up carrots and celery. When I feel kinda nibbly, and open the fridge, there they are, staring me in the face. Otherwise, I'm going to grab the easiest thing—which is probably also the least healthy. We're designed to choose the path of least resistance. It's in our genetic code and has helped us survive as a species.

You have to be a good parent to yourself. It takes a little bit of work to be optimally healthy. Suck it up, sunshine. Once you feel the benefits, the action is reinforced. For example, I'm very lazy in the morning. It's not my best time. So I put green veggies in the blender the night before and stow it in the fridge. All I have to do in the morning is hit the on button, pour the smoothie in a Mason jar, and I'm ready to go. This is something any woman can do, whether she works outside the home or not. It takes me about three minutes, but I'd never do it if I didn't prepare the fixings the night before.

Supplementation for Maintenance

Nobody wants to continue taking all the vitamins and herbs in the 30-Day Plan forever. And I don't expect you to. The 30-Day Plan is a program designed to treat, boost, and balance hormones. Adrenal fatigue is the one thing that can take longer to respond. Some people benefit from taking adrenal supplements for up to three months or more. This is because our cells can live for up to three months. And we want to ensure that new cells that make our hormones are nourished sufficiently to do the job.

Take TestoGain (described below) for as long as you want a vibrant life. You can stop if you want to. But we live in a society that depletes our hormones before our life span ends, so the two no longer match. We're depleting our hormones at a much earlier stage than we did in the past because of how we live our lives. If you're afraid hot flashes and other symptoms may return, continue the herbs that help for as long as necessary.

If you scored low on the estrogen quiz, you can take all the supplements that I recommend for thirty days and then begin taking EstroMend (Douglas Laboratories) or Hormone Balance (Vital Nutrients).

For testosterone, I recommend using topical TestoGain, a testosterone formula made by Integrative Therapeutics, and maca. Testosterone is the secret to aging vibrantly, and we want to boost it naturally and continuously to help our bodies, our brains, and our lives. Also see my thirty day vitamin packs for a shortcut.

Sleep Better Forever

There are five things I want you to pay attention to regarding sleep in order to sleep well and wake rejuvenated.

1. Create a sleep-hygiene routine. This is a term used in medicine and has nothing to do with going to bed clean. It describes the routine and pattern of our behavior, our surroundings, and the time we go to bed. Have you ever noticed that babies start to yawn and rub their eyes during their nighttime routine? I used to bathe my girls at night when they were babies and then massage them with coconut oil while we listened to music. They would rub their eyes and get sleepier and sleepier as their bodies sank into slumber. We are no different. Our bodies need a routine to tell our brains that it is time for the day to be done and for sleep to start.

Start getting ready for bed at least twenty to thirty minutes before you need to be asleep. Studies show that turning off iPads, computers, phones, and TV for one or two hours before bed has a positive effect on the quality and quantity of sleep. Use a wonderful facial moisturizer after cleaning your skin, and don't forget your neck and lips. If you especially love scents, lavender has been shown to be wonderful for inducing sleep. Get a linen spray and spray your room or linen before getting into bed.

2. Ensure that your room is dark, or wear a sleeping mask.

3. Control noise. Many people find that white noise is very restful. Many of us do not have a home that is completely silent all night long. A fan on low (turned away from you) can drown out any early morning sounds of traffic or neighbors and help keep us asleep.

4. Turn off cortisol. The supplement Cortisol Manager (Integrative Therapeutics) is an amazing way to tell your adrenals, "Shh, it's time to go to sleep now."

5. Turn on the relaxation response. Use meditation, breathing exercises, or listen to the Holosync.

If you have recurring sleep problems, continue to use over-the-counter progesterone cream as directed on the bottle. Some women need more, but this is a good place to start.

Titrate Melatonin

Another answer for many people is over-the-counter melatonin. There are several advantages to having healthy melatonin levels. Taken at night, melatonin dramatically enhances your immune system. It is one of the most powerful antioxidants, and it reduces your risk of many cancers. It also helps you get a restful night's sleep. You will fall asleep promptly, and experience fitting and realistic dreams. (As we age, our dreams become less frequent and less realistic. Many older people are completely unaware of dreaming at all.)

Melatonin allows you to be aware that you were dreaming if you wake during the night. When you open your eyes in the morning, you will feel refreshed and ready for the new day.

The proper dose of melatonin varies from person to person.

Some of my patients in their forties can't tolerate even 1 mg. On the other hand, most people in their fifties, sixties, and above require higher doses.

1. Take 1 mg of melatonin shortly before bedtime.
2. Continue for three consecutive nights and observe your reaction.
3. Increase the dose by 1 mg every three days. Keep this up until you find that you fall asleep promptly, have realistic dreams, and awaken rested and refreshed the next morning.
4. Realize that some people could require up to 12 mg of melatonin per night.

Dosages of 1 mg and 3 mg are available in health-food stores and drugstores, as well as an extended release form for people who fall asleep easily but wake in the middle of the night.

Note, however, that melatonin works best in a pitch-dark room. It won't be produced and released optimally if you have a clock radio that lights up or a smoke detector with a neon light, or if you don't have blackout curtains.

Sleep issues are much too important to your health and well-being to ignore them or automatically pop a prescription sleeping pill. We know that nurses who work the night shift have higher breast-cancer rates than nurses who work days. We think it has something to do with the fact that the body naturally releases melatonin at night. Shift work and sleeping during the day may result in less melatonin being released.

Improve Breathing and Meditation Skills and Expand Your Repertoire

You're learning to change your attitudes and your behavior, but you can't take control of your life unless you handle stress as well. There are many forms of meditation to help accomplish that, such as moving meditation (like tai chi) and Transcendental Meditation, which

ENERGY/VITALITY CHECKUP

A good start is only half the battle. The big question is: Can you keep the gains you've worked so hard for and even tweak areas that need more attention? To monitor how you're doing, take this self-test every three to six months. The results will help you recognize signs that you're back-sliding into your old ways.

I often (write down the score for your answer):

	AGREE (2)	AGREE SOMEWHAT (1)	DISAGREE (0)
1. Lose my sense of humor/take life too seriously.	____	____	____
2. Experience doubt or indecision.	____	____	____
3. Feel worried or anxious.	____	____	____
4. Feel overcautious or pessimistic.	____	____	____
5. Lack self-confidence or feel low self-esteem.	____	____	____
6. Feel stressed or tense.	____	____	____
7. Feel irritable or oversensitive.	____	____	____
8. Have a hard time concentrating and thinking clearly.	____	____	____
9. Feel fatigued.	____	____	____
10. Use coffee, tobacco, sugar, or other stimulants as a pick-me-up.	____	____	____
11. Experience nervous indigestion.	____	____	____
12. Lose my sex drive.	____	____	____
13. Have sleep problems.	____	____	____
14. Feel more tired in the morning than at bedtime.	____	____	____

15. Feel run-down.   ___   ___   ___

16. Feel depressed.   ___   ___   ___

17. Want to cry for no reason.   ___   ___   ___

18. If I relax and am not busy, I
    feel exhausted.   ___   ___   ___

19. Have difficulty expressing my
    feelings.   ___   ___   ___

20. Experience rapid heartbeat or
    panic.   ___   ___   ___

21. Feel moody.   ___   ___   ___

22. Wonder whether life is worth
    living or feel suicidal.   ___   ___   ___

23. Worry about not having
    enough money.   ___   ___   ___

24. Fear health problems.   ___   ___   ___

25. Fear criticism.   ___   ___   ___

26. Fear loss of love.   ___   ___   ___

27. Fear old age or death.   ___   ___   ___

28. Feel "Something is the matter
    with me, but I don't know
    what."   ___   ___   ___

29. Think I might be "losing it" or
    "going crazy."   ___   ___   ___

Total Score: ___

0–25: High Vitality

26–40: Good Vitality

41–55: Average Vitality

56–70: Low Vitality

71 and Above: Burnout

is the most scientifically studied and proven form of meditation in the world. Listening to guided meditation is another option. Pick the form you like best, because then you'll do it. Yet you should also have more than one kind up your sleeve as a backup. If you rely only on tai chi, what do you do when you're not in a convenient place for it? If you do Transcendental Meditation, which requires a quiet room, and you're traveling, you should have a guided meditation to use. Be prepared for the unexpected curveballs that life throws at you.

I spent time learning Transcendental Meditation, yet I was shocked to find that I do not have twenty minutes of absolute solitude in my life most days. Some people can meditate in their car, but I was too self-conscious. My meditation practice now includes TM when I can, and my husband and I listen to the Holosync every night as we fall asleep. The change I noticed is significant. It feels as if I have more space between the moments in my day, and I am able to focus on gratitude instead of on what is missing or isn't perfect.

Incidentally, belly breathing (see page 80) is a form of meditation. Remember, it shifts your body into the parasympathetic nervous system. It's been shown to lower blood pressure, relieve headaches and stomach issues, decrease depression, calm anxiety, and more. The diaphragm contracts and actually allows the lungs to fill with air, because it creates a negative pressure. It pulls the lungs down. If you're at work or elsewhere where it's inconvenient to lie down to do it, you can graduate to a chair. Imagine a travel scenario, for example, where you're waiting for a flight departure near the boarding gate. Just loosen your pants or skirt before you sit down, and make sure you consciously focus on feeling your belly expand. It's an instant switch to concentrating on the here and now. Lying on the floor is simply the easiest position for breathing because you're totally relaxed, don't have anything to think about, and aren't using any muscles to sit. Actually, you can do the same once you're on the plane.

In a way, belly breathing reminds me of a yoga pose called Shavasana. You lie on your back with legs apart and arms by your side and away from your body, with your palms up. It's sometimes called the dead man's pose, since your eyes are closed. Considered one of the key parts of yoga, Shavasana allows the body to reset itself and induces deep muscle relaxation. It's a very powerful position to be in, but it isn't always convenient.

The more you incorporate belly breathing into your life, the more your body will "remember" to do it throughout the day. Belly breathing is actually one of the best preventive medicines you can use. In the parasympathetic nervous system, your body sends out "soldier cells" that look for trouble, such as cancer. The body basically kills these abnormal cells through a process called apoptosis, which is programmed cellular death. Belly breathing is one of the ways to head off early cancer and inflammation, and heal injuries.

Move Your Body

Most people don't start the day with meditation or exercise of any kind. If they do exercise in the morning, it's something they rush to check off their list, rather than an activity they engage in with full presence and enjoyment.

In my clinic we have a 3-2-1 challenge. It is a 14-day challenge to walk thirty minutes a day, meditate for ten minutes twice a day, and have one green juice or smoothie a day. I give my patients a free massage for accomplishing this and sharing their experiences.

One of my patients, Susan, said the challenge made her realize that small changes could really add up. She lost five pounds in the fourteen days and had a burst of energy. Beth was reluctant to join the challenge. She felt that she could walk at lunchtime and find time to breathe or meditate for ten minutes, but she couldn't see herself doing the juice or smoothie part. We discussed the benefits of these drinks, and she felt so overwhelmed and tired that she was willing to trust me and try it. Beth now says green smoothies are the one constant in her day.

Patients have taken this idea to their workplace, and large and small corporations have created similar challenges to improve employee health. I urge you to be a leader in health and vitality. When those around you share similar principles, it will be even easier to stay on track.

I pay my employees for two hours per week to meditate and exercise. We use the honor system when reporting this time. I want to encourage my staff to implement activities that I know will make them healthier and happier.

Sitting Is the New Smoking

A lot of research out of Harvard, the Mayo Clinic, and elsewhere has linked too much sitting with an increased risk of death (especially for the obese and people who have metabolic syndrome, which is characterized by high blood pressure, high cholesterol and sugar, and excess body fat around the waist). In studies, working out after sitting doesn't seem to undo the effects of being sedentary. This is very scary in a world where we do everything from a seated position—work, watching TV, and driving.

A new 2014 Cornell study of 92,234 menopausal and postmenopausal women ages fifty to seventy-nine, published online, adds to the literature. The research found that women with more than eleven hours of sedentary time per day had a 12 percent increase in premature, all-cause mortality when compared with women with inactive time of four hours or fewer. The most sedentary group also boosted the risk of death from cardiovascular disease by 13 percent, coronary heart disease by 27 percent, and cancer by 21 percent. The author noted that too much sedentary time made it harder to regain strength and physical function.

Earlier research by the American Cancer Society found that women who sat for more than six hours a day were 94 percent more likely to die than their more active counterparts.

My recommendations are:

1. Move more throughout your day. Stand when you answer the phone. Remind yourself to get up and walk around more after prolonged sitting. (Posting reminder notes on your computer or desk can help.) Get into the habit of rising from the couch and walking (to the bathroom, if necessary) anytime commercials interrupt a television program you're watching.

2. Get a standing desk. People balk at this idea because they feel they'll be less productive and more fatigued. But a variety of sit/stand desks (which allow you to do both) is available online today at a wide range of prices. To check them out, just use your search engine.

Recognize What Testosterone and Hormone Balance Can't Do

I wish balancing your hormones could solve all your problems. But the reality is that hormones are not always the only thing contributing to your health issues. For example, some women can't lose weight due to food allergies. They absorb sugar and simple carbohydrates (which are bad for you) quickly and easily due to inflammation in the gut—and have trouble absorbing the amino acids from protein, as well as vitamins and minerals. As a result, the body still isn't satisfied with the nutrition it receives. You feel hungry, so you eat more. If you don't lose as much weight as you want on the 30-Day Plan, you may be allergic or sensitive to some foods without realizing it. We are not all allergic or sensitive to the same things. Though I think that the gluten and wheat products today do not resemble those of our grandparents' time, and many people feel better not eating them, gluten sensitivity is not the same as a true allergy. After doing thousands of food-sensitivity blood tests for patients, I've found that no two people are exactly the same.

My patient Kelly, an attractive fifty-year-old commercial real-estate agent, walked into my office one day weighing 165 pounds. She was five-three (not nearly tall enough to carry all that weight). Despite many attempts to slim down, she had been unsuccessful.

I suspected that Kelly had food allergies, and took some tests. The results showed that she had an allergy to dairy that she'd never been aware of. She had yogurt every morning, thinking it was a healthier option than cereal or toast. In fact, you can be allergic to the sugar part of dairy, the protein part, or to both. And more than six hundred thousand Americans have such allergies—according to the American College of Allergy, Asthma & Immunology. Although children usually outgrow the allergy, it does persist in some adults.

I took Kelly off dairy, but dairy turns up in a lot of unexpected foods that are processed. What Kelly needed was fresh vegetables and a lot more protein. I customized a nonprescription program to heal her gut, which included L-Glutamine, probiotics, and Blue Heron, a supplement that is a combination of many herbs that heal the gut, such as slippery elm and fenugreek. She also took chewable enzymes to help her digestion.

She changed her way of eating and respected her sensitivities—and lost ten pounds in one month—and did it without a diet.

Low Libido

From time to time I ask my patients, "How is your libido, and are you satisfied with where it's at?" They often say it's low. And I ask, "How is it when you're on holiday and you have no responsibilities?" If they respond, "Fine," I tell them, "I can help you, but not with hormones. That's a time-management and stress issue. It has nothing to do with your hormones."

The point is that testosterone increases your desire to have sex and improves the quality of the actual sexual experience. But sex is not just about your hormones. You may want to blame it on that, but it's a bad rap. Time management of your sex life is about staying connected, making each other a priority, and about being grateful every single day for one solid thing about your spouse. Sex is often the thing that happens after everything else, with whatever energy you have left. Women especially need to feel energized (not exhausted) to want and enjoy sex. Try to schedule intercourse with your spouse at a different time of day. Take a morning shower together, head to the bedroom after dinner or right after the kids go to bed, rather than waiting until 10 or 11 p.m.

It's a whole mind shift. There's a lot out in books, magazines, and online about making your sex life sizzle by using testosterone. The reality is that if you're up at 6 a.m. and go to bed at 11 p.m. and work full-time, it doesn't matter how much hormone balance you have. You're exhausted and just want to hug your pillow. We must put the important things in our lives first. Sex can be an amazing part of a healthy relationship. If you and your partner want to increase your desire and enjoyment in this area, make it a priority. It may not seem sexy to have an appointment for intimacy. But I assure you that the sex will improve if you create a time for it when you are both energetic and able to enjoy the experience.

Why You Fall Off the Nutrition Wagon

Do you know anyone who *hasn't* slipped off a diet? I don't. But there are ways to help yourself when it happens. The first step is to identify the reason it occurs. I find that there are five main causes: (1) cravings (urgent desire for certain foods); (2) compulsive eating (an irresistible urge to eat, especially against your conscious wishes); (3) sadness or depression; (4) anxiety; and (5) impulsive eating (eating without forethought). In the latter case, you sit at the movies and eat an entire bag of popcorn. You keep reaching for the popcorn without thinking, and now it's gone.

Is your answer yes to one (or more) of these? Here are some quick solutions:

1. Get your cravings under control.
✧ Keep your blood sugar balanced.
✧ Try alpha lipoic acid.
✧ Chromium picolinate helps reduce sugar cravings.
✧ N-acetyl cysteine helps reduce compulsive cravings.
✧ Eat protein at breakfast.

2. If you are a compulsive/impulsive eater, try:
✧ Exercise
✧ 5-HTP
✧ Saint John's-Wort

3. If you eat when sad or depressed, these may help:
✧ Fish oil
✧ Vitamin D
✧ Sam-E
✧ Exercise

4. If you eat when anxious, these may help:
✧ Meditation
✧ Vitamin B6
✧ Magnesium
✧ GABA

5. If you are an impulsive eater (reach for food without thinking, easily distracted), these may help:
✧ Increased protein in diet
✧ L-tyrosine

CHAPTER 11

When Women Need More— Bioidentical Hormones

The medical community intervenes with heart disease and diabetes in this country, but not with hormone problems. Yes, it's true that plenty of women are treated for hormone issues. When women go to the doctor complaining of severe hot flashes, night sweats that drench the sheets, vaginal dryness that causes painful intercourse, or have had a hysterectomy, they receive hormones. But that's when they have obvious problems that everyone can see. It's different, however, when women in their forties start experiencing mild anxiety, depression, brain fog, sleep problems, and difficulty losing those ten to fifteen pounds. These women don't receive a hormone evaluation. Their symptoms are treated with an anti-anxiety medication, an antidepressant, and/or a sleeping pill. The prescription pad comes out unless you have full-blown symptoms of hormone deficiency.

The flashes and sweats that are normally thought of as menopausal occur when the car has completely run out of gas (hormones). But that's not when the problem started. It started ten years earlier. You're not running on all cylinders when your tank is only half full of hormones. Many symptoms you're experiencing that may be attributed to psychiatric or other conditions are likely the result of a hormone imbalance. Why wait for appropriate treatment when help is available now?

We don't wait until you have a stroke to address your blood

pressure. A stroke is the end result of high blood pressure, in many cases. We keep lowering the recommended number when your blood pressure should be treated, and we intervene earlier and earlier. We keep lowering the number your blood sugar should be and intervene earlier and earlier. I want women to wake up and realize that their hormones should be treated the same way.

Everybody thinks that our hormone levels are down because we're aging. But we're aging because our hormone levels decline. We age more rapidly when our hormones are out of whack. Every woman can attest to this by looking in the mirror. Sagging skin, wrinkles, extra weight, lack of tone in muscles in the arms and legs— all of these change at a much more rapid rate from the midforties to the midsixties than at any other decade in our lives.

Even if hormone imbalance is treated, it is often not addressed in a holistic, naturopathic, integrated approach to how you supplement, eat, move, and think. I believe it's time to change that. I've seen people in their forties and fifties with hormone levels and deficiencies I'd expect to see in their sixties and seventies. How do you know if you need prescription help? If you don't get results from the 30-Day Plan, you may be a candidate for bioidentical hormones. If you get results, but want more, you're also a candidate. So are women with specific health issues, such as severe osteoporosis or significant adrenal fatigue. Testosterone levels are sometimes so low—and estrogen and progesterone imbalance so rampant—that it may take more than over-the-counter supplements, nutrition, and lifestyle changes to help. In either of these cases, you will need to consult a physician.

Women who must undergo a hysterectomy (or have already done so) are also candidates. Studies show that having a hysterectomy puts women into full-blown menopause earlier. Even if the ovaries are retained, hormone deficiencies and imbalances can be quite significant in these women. I treat such patients with bioidentical hormones by prescription in Seattle and all over the United States via Skype and phone appointments.

What's a Bioidentical Hormone?

As the name implies, bioidentical hormones are the same as your body's own natural hormones—and are created by compounding pharmacies or manufacturers to mimic Mother Nature. The first prescription for bioidentical hormones was written thirty-five years ago by my friend Dr. Jonathan Wright. In contrast, synthetic hormones neither look nor act like your own hormones. The synthetic estrogen Premarin, which millions of women used to take for estrogen replacement, is made from the urine of a pregnant mare. And I've told you how your body reacts to foreign substances. Other synthetic hormones also contain substances the body cannot recognize.

Synthetic hormones are also taken by mouth, so your liver has to metabolize them. This increases the risk of blood clots, because the liver is not equipped to process hormones from the GI tract. Estrogen of any kind should not be taken by mouth.

Background on the Hormone Controversy

Some of the decisions women make about hormones and the fear they have about hormone use comes from the results of the Women's Health Initiative. The Women's Health Initiative was a fifteen-year study created to investigate the most common causes of death, disability, and a decrease in quality of life in postmenopausal women. This enormous clinical trial included 161,808 women and studied synthetic estrogen with and without progestin (synthetic progesterone). The shocking results showed a statistically significant increase in coronary heart disease, stroke, cardiovascular disease, pulmonary embolism (lung clots), and breast cancer.

These results led the National Heart, Lung, and Blood Institute (NHLBI) to stop the trial early in 2002. Tens of thousands of women abruptly halted their synthetic-hormone-replacement therapy.

The downside of synthetic hormones is not news for those of us who practice natural medicine. We can outline many ways in which synthetic hormones result in increased health risks for very serious conditions.

Bioidentical hormones have been prescribed for more than three decades, and studied in depth. To date, studies do not show a direct link between bioidentical hormones and cancer, clots, or heart disease. There are important facts, however, that you and your health provider should know if you take bioidentical hormones. For example, testosterone can be converted into bad estrogen. If you take bioidentical hormones, your estrogen levels should be checked. The best test for this is a urine test, which will ensure that your body is not converting testosterone (or even estrogen) into bad (cancer-causing) estrogen. If this conversion occurs, there are many ways to fix it. But not if you don't know that it's happening! Your doctor is there to help you. If you feel you are not being listened to or do not have a good relationship with him/her, find another doctor. You are allowed to fire your doctor. I'll show you how on page 243 in Chapter 12.

The research supports the safe use of bioidenticals. I prefer low-dose forms of bioidentical testosterone and estrogen that are cream-based to allow dermal (through the skin) penetration without increasing the risk of blood clots. There are also patches, injectable forms, and troches (medicated lozenges that melt in the buccal mucosa of your mouth). Progesterone is the only hormone that is safe in pill form, because it doesn't pass through the liver. Therefore it's not in danger of being converted into unsafe metabolites.

Life-Changing Results from Testosterone Replacement Today

Testosterone optimization is truly a secret weapon for women as they age. But too much testosterone can result in increased facial hair, acne, and other side effects. The word "testosterone" alone is often enough to frighten women. But we now know that those side effects need never happen—and that women require only a fraction of the dosage men receive to get life-changing results. Low dosage virtually eliminates testosterone's objectionable side effects. And, if you are simply boosting your own testosterone without a prescription, it is very unlikely that your body will produce too much, because it needed help in the first place.

I treat patients who need more than nonprescription help with bioidentical testosterone replacement every day in my clinic. Women who come to me with osteoporosis, severe depression, and other symptoms benefit greatly from prescription testosterone. I start with 1 or 2 mg and slowly raise the dosage to a maximum of 5 mg. This dosage replaces only the testosterone that has been lost. Nothing more. A small amount can make a big difference for women, and side effects are extremely rare with low doses. In the small percentage of cases where side effects do occur, these effects disappear as soon as the testosterone is stopped and restarted at a lower dose. The side effects do not return.

Another concern expressed at times is that studies of long-term testosterone use have been done mostly in men. However, that's true of most long-term pharmaceutical studies, although the assumption is that the results apply to women, too. The blood-pressure medication that you may be taking was not studied on a women-only group, yet the benefits are assumed to apply to both men and women.

There is no FDA-approved testosterone for women. As a result, compounding pharmacies are the source for this prescription. Because testosterone builds bone, I offer bioidentical testosterone to all women who have been given a diagnosis of osteopenia or osteoporosis. The traditional treatment for these conditions, Fosamax, has frightening side effects, such as bone loss in the jaw. A May 2012 article in *Menopausal Medicine*, the journal of the American Society for Reproductive Medicine, reviewed research on why testosterone might be prescribed for women in low doses and made a strong case for its multiple therapeutic benefits. The article found no evidence that testosterone causes heart disease or that past use of low-dose testosterone increases the risk of breast cancer.

The testosterone I prescribe for most of my patients is a topical cream applied once a day, every day, preferably in the morning. Injectable forms of testosterone are available, but they are usually in the much higher dosage used for men. In addition, the dose of an injection creates peaks and valleys. But a cream's pattern is like a gently rolling hill that rises slightly and declines slightly throughout the day. Because the cream involves everyday dosage, it's also much more controlled and natural than an injection.

The best place to put the cream is the part of the body where it's going to be most easily absorbed. That is on a mucous membrane, which exists in four places: the eyes, and inside the mouth, nose, and vagina. The latter is the best location—either on the inner parts of the labia majora (the larger, outer vaginal lips) or in the vaginal vault (where you insert a tampon). An alternative location is the lower inner part of the arm. Yes, the cream may rub off on your husband, so it is best to use it after sex or when you are not going to be intimate. Caution: To ensure that your testosterone does not transfer to children or animals, apply it to an area that is covered, or at a time when you will not touch others. I don't recommended using testosterone or any other hormone cream on your breasts or under the arm.

Incidentally, lots of media attention has focused on testosterone lately—most recently, on the connection between testosterone replacement and heart disease. We have known for many years that replacing testosterone by prescription without balancing other hormones can lead to plaque formation and heart disease. That is one of the many reasons that all the hormones need to be balanced together.

Bioidentical Estrogen

There is currently a big discussion in the medical community about the difference between bioidentical hormones and synthetic hormones. Shockingly, despite all the evidence in the Women's Health Initiative study that showed synthetic estrogens do no good and actually cause great harm, these old estrogens that our mothers used are again being prescribed to some women. Doctors abruptly took women off synthetic estrogen after the WHI study was stopped. But they're now slowly putting some patients back on these estrogens. Justifications I've heard from patients include: "My doctor says it's a smaller dose, so it won't harm me." My response is: A smaller dose of something harmful is still harmful. And there are no studies showing that the harm done by synthetic estrogen was dose-related. The problem with these hormones is the way they are metabolized—and they're not recognized by our bodies, because they're completely foreign substances.

Today, both bioidentical and synthetic estrogen are available to women who need help, and there are options for patches and creams in varying doses. I have helped thousands of women overcome hot flashes, painful intercourse, and more by prescribing bioidentical estrogen as part of a holistic, comprehensive hormone plan. Remember, there are three common estrogens: estriol, estrone, and estradiol. Estradiol and estriol disappear when we get older to a greater degree than estrone does. Therefore, we replace them. The estrogen bioidentical hormone is called Biest (as in "two estrogens"), a topical cream available by prescription. As with testosterone cream, the best place to apply the estrogen cream is the place that's going to have the most absorption—and that is on the vaginal mucosa.

We used to prescribe Triest, which was "three estrogens," the three found in women. But we've learned over the years that women have the highest levels of estrone, which is kind of the "bad guy," as we get older. More estrone isn't needed to create balance. What women need is estradiol and estriol.

There's another advantage to the vaginal location. If you experience discomfort during sex, it may not (as commonly believed) be caused just by a lack of lubrication. The problem is that the vaginal tissue thins, like rice paper. It's very fragile, and it rips during sex. Women tell me, "Sex still hurts, even when I use a lubricant." However, estrogen cream, applied in the vagina, actually rebuilds the tissue and restores it to health. Sex doesn't hurt anymore.

Some women don't want to put cream in their vagina. In that case, I move to the next best option. I tell them to apply it on the lower part of their inner arm (above the wrist), and spread it from there to the elbow. The elbow has the least amount of fat, and the goal is to avoid absorption by fat. If your estrogen becomes trapped in fat, it cannot travel in the bloodstream and create its benefits all over the body. Estrogen cream reduces hot flashes, night sweats, brain fog—all the symptoms mentioned in the estrogen self-test.

My patients take anywhere from ½ mg to 3 mg or 3½ mg of Biest cream. On Days 1–25, you receive a full dose and stop for the remainder of the month. For some women, this "off" time results in hot flashes and a return of all the things they were seeking to fix in the first place. In that instance, we switch to a half dose for the rest of the month. I want to give the smallest amount needed to optimize the hormones, even though Biest is a bioidentical. My philosophy is: "Let's not take your levels back to those of a twenty-nine-year-old. You're not twenty-nine. Let's take them to an optimal level for where you're at."

Bioidentical estrogen is approved by the FDA. Dosage should create natural estrogen levels via timing. We were never intended to have the exact same dose of estrogen every single day. That is why I am not a fan of estrogen pellets, which secrete estrogen all day, every day. There is a natural rise and fall in estrogen and progesterone. When the levels of both fall, there is a period. We must respect and try to fine-tune estrogen and progesterone dosage to produce that same rhythm. As a result, a very small percentage of women who take bioidenticals (maybe 1 percent or 2 percent), who are way past their last period and into menopause, have a period.

In my clinic, I tell everyone who starts hormone therapy about the possibility of a period ahead of time in order to head off cancer fears. We've all been warned that bleeding after menopause can be a sign of ovarian or uterine cancer. Thousands of biopsies, which are very painful, are performed for that reason. So every patient of mine gets one free bleed if that happens when she begins bioidentical hormone-replacement therapy (BHRT)—and then I make adjustments. My goal is not to have women in their sixties have a menstrual cycle. I do know that some practitioners deliberately bring on a regular period, because there are women who actually want it (in the mistaken belief that it's an anti-aging measure).

The fact is, there is no such thing as anti-aging. You are getting older every single day. Don't try to fight it; finesse it. Make getting older graceful and full of wonder and health and vitality. As long as you have your energy, it's kind of nice to age with the wisdom you've gained. I always say that I don't mind looking my age as long as I look great for my age!

How About Patches?

There is no testosterone patch that's readily available for women. The doses are too high for us. But there are estrogen patches. A common one is called the Vivelle-Dot. Although this is bioidentical estradiol, it is only estradiol, which is one step away from truly mimicking nature as much as we can.

The problem with estrogen patches is that they're available only in set, manufactured dosages. You pick the one that's closest to what you need. This is a prime example of the one-size-fits-all mentality of Western medicine.

Patches also make it harder to create the desired rise-and-fall cycle. Cutting the patch for a smaller dose inhibits its slow-release capacity. I have some patients who need half a patch at the end of the month instead of stopping completely, and not all patches can be cut. In contrast, a bioidentical hormone prescription is customized to the exact dose required for your frame, height and weight, your symptoms, and your blood levels—not the closest manufactured dose.

Nevertheless, some patients just say, "I'm not going to use a cream every day," and choose a patch. Part of medicine is about meeting patients where they're at. The patch may also protect the heart, according to the results of a review of the data from the Women's Health Initiative published, in 2014, in the journal *Menopause*. The observational study compared different doses and delivery methods. Researchers concluded that bioidentical estradiol and the estrogen patch in smaller doses may create a lower risk of heart attack and stroke than estrogen pills.

Bioidentical Progesterone

Estrogen can't be addressed without addressing progesterone, which women can take in cream or pill form, or both. Progesterone is one of the few hormones we can safely take by mouth, and there's actually an advantage to that. When taken by mouth, progesterone crosses the blood-brain barrier and enhances sleep and reduces anxiety, while stimulating the GABA receptors, whose natural function is to reduce anxiety and help us feel calm. I let my patients decide which form to use, because the difference isn't huge. About half say, "I'm already doing cream estrogen, so I'll do cream." The other half respond, "No, cream is too messy. I'll just pop a pill at my bedside." Another set of women experience too much of a drop in their progesterone levels when they stop using the progesterone cream. We do a low-dose pill every night as a safety net to prevent this dip.

As with estrogen cream, the best place for absorption of progesterone cream is the vaginal mucosa. And the best time for application is at night, because progesterone helps you sleep.

Cream users who no longer have a period opt for progesterone cream on Days 11–25 of the month. The most significant impulse for your body to have a period is called the progesterone withdrawal. The body sees progesterone, and then it's taken away—which is the signal for a period. If a woman still has periods, she stops taking progesterone when bleeding begins.

Testosterone is not produced in a rise-and-fall fashion. That's why most women who need testosterone replacement take from 1 mg to 5 mg of testosterone cream daily (at any time of the day).

Hormone Replacement for Hysterectomy

Hysterectomy is known as "surgical menopause." This procedure surgically removes the uterus, and sometimes the cervix and/or ovaries and Fallopian tubes—and actually hijacks your body. Who you were and how you used to feel have been snatched away from you. Cognition, memory, and sexuality may decline. Depression or a sense of loss is common, depending on what has been removed. You have also started an accelerated menopause, even if you still have your ovaries. When Marian, a fifty-three-year-old stockbroker, came to see me, she was distraught about her lagging recovery from a hysterectomy. She told me, "I don't understand it. I thought I'd bounce back from this surgery, and I'm not doing that." She was tired all the time, bloated, and cranky. And I said, "You've just been robbed." Her response was, "That's exactly how I feel."

Marian's ob-gyn had put her on the usual estrogen and progesterone post-surgery. I recommended switching her to bioidentical versions—and I added testosterone. Marian felt better at her one-month follow-up, but not great. After I questioned her, she admitted that she had been using the estrogen and the progesterone but was reluctant to use the testosterone. I reassured her that the 1 mg dose was far below doses that create side effects—and explained all the benefits for her energy level, figure, bones, and brain that testosterone would provide. This time she promised to try it. On her return visit a month later, she reported that adding testosterone truly made a difference in getting her life back. She loved how she looked, and she felt great.

Post-hysterectomy, some women are put on estrogen alone. And every physician learned in medical school that you do not give estrogen by itself. (It's called unopposed estrogen.) Estrogen alone has been indisputably proven to increase the risk of uterine cancer. The excuse given by physicians for prescribing estrogen only is "My patients no longer have a uterus." The problem is you have estrogen receptors throughout your body—in your brain, your breasts, everywhere—that are balanced and tempered by the progesterone and testosterone receptors in the same places. Our hormones work together, in all parts of our bodies.

Research findings presented in 2013 at the American Academy of Neurology revealed that the younger a woman is when she has surgical menopause, the faster cognition and memory decline. In the study of approximately 1,800 postmenopausal women, hormone-replacement therapy slowed declines in those who received it. The results are critically important for women's quality of life, because an estimated twenty million women in the United States have had a hysterectomy, and about six hundred thousand hysterectomies are performed annually in this country. According to the Centers for Disease Control (CDC), hysterectomy is topped only by Cesarean section as the most frequently performed surgery for women of reproductive age in the United States.

As Marian discovered, testosterone can improve your sex life, too. Research published in the May 2005 issue of *Obstetrics and Gynecology,* the official publication of the American College of Obstetricians and Gynecologists, confirms this. The double-blind, placebo-controlled six-month trial followed 533 women with hypoactive-sexual-desire disorder who had previous hysterectomies and bilateral oophorectomy (removal of both ovaries). The researchers found that the group that received a 300 mcg testosterone patch twice a week had a significant improvement in satisfying sexual activity and sexual desire, compared with the placebo group, along with a drop in personal distress. The patch was well tolerated.

Small Changes with Big Payoffs

I look at patients' past medical conditions, and I give them bioidentical testosterone, estrogen, and progesterone if they've had a hysterectomy. I prescribe testosterone for osteoporosis, along with a little extra progesterone, because it stimulates cells that build bone. I also add a little estrogen, because it makes the collagen that knits bones together well. It's much better to do that than to use Fosamax, which has scary side effects.

I also use bioidentical hormones to treat conditions like severe adrenal fatigue. It's going to take six months to two years for adrenal patients to heal. I want to increase their quality of life right now and take the pressure off the adrenal glands.

As for thyroid hormones, they are available in good synthetic forms, and may help you function better if you're hypothyroid (below optimal). Many people are treated with the medication Synthroid (sometimes also known as levothyroxine). Synthroid contains synthetic T4, which is the same as that produced in the thyroid gland. If your body has a problem converting T4 to T3 because of a sluggish liver (90 percent of the conversion takes place in the liver), T4 won't help you feel better. But I have patients whose primary-care doctors offer resistance to raising their medication. However, physicians don't have to worry, because people don't feel well when they take too much thyroid medication—and it can quickly be scaled back. The idea is to start low and raise medication slowly to avoid overtreating. Lots of women would love their doctors to be more assertive in treating thyroid problems.

Boosting and balancing with bioidentical hormone medication when necessary is a complicated business. But it's been proven to be safe. Compounding pharmacies are essential, because one size doesn't fit all. These pharmacies are certified by the PCAB (Pharmacy Compounding Accreditation Board), and you can look up certified pharmacies in each state on the PCAB website, www.pcab.org.

Even a few basic changes can vastly improve your quality of life.

CHAPTER 12

Living Fully for the Rest of Your Life

When we were younger, we opened our eyes in the morning, sunlight hit our retinas and was converted into serotonin, and we said, "I'm going to ride my bike today." Now we say "ugh" and hit the snooze alarm. Later on, it takes one or two cups of coffee to make us feel alive. But, hopefully, that scenario is already changing for you. You know it is possible to be leaner, stronger, calmer, and sharper. You can feel a difference in your energy level and in the quality of your sleep.

But this is a tough world we live in today. We're exposed to more and more toxins and to unending stress, which affect our testosterone and other hormone levels. For ourselves and for our loved ones, we can create a new environment by raising our awareness and taking sensible protective measures.

The Case for Eating Organic

Although vitamins and minerals can be a great way to improve the micronutrient content of your diet, the very best way to get nutrients is from food. I'm talking about food grown without pesticides and chemical fertilizers. But we now know that the vitamins contained in plant-based foods are only part of the picture. A bigger and possibly even more important part is phytonutrients. These are chemicals that plants produce for protection from germs, fungi, bugs, and other damaging threats. So far, twenty-five thousand phytonutrients have been identified. Many experts suggest that eating or drinking phytonutrients can prevent disease and help maintain optimal health. For example, brightly colored vegetables, such as green, red, and yellow peppers and eggplants, are jam-packed with phytonutrients.

The question is, do plants grown with pesticides or genetically modified to be resistant to bugs and disease still produce the same quantity and quality of phytonutrients? You may say, "Okay, I am going to eat organically grown, nongenetically modified fruits and vegetables." Yet you sit down in November to enjoy a fresh mango flown in from Chile. This mango had to be picked well before it was ripe in order to survive long enough to be shipped thousands of miles away—and sit in the produce section of the supermarket to be sold.

Has the mango lost phytonutrient content along the way? If the mango was picked when green, has it had time to develop all the phytonutrients nature intended? We'll probably never know the answers to these questions, because there are no studies, and backing to finance research isn't available. My policy is to use common sense and realize that the answers are likely to be no. Therefore, eat organic and eat local. Your farmers' market, or a local farmer who delivers to your door, is a great way to ensure that you get the full complement of phytonutrients. Fight the free radicals associated with cancer with farm products grown locally in the dirt and sun until ripe. Prevent and treat diseases with "farm-acy" instead of pharmacy as much as possible.

The imported produce found in the grocery store even lacks a smell, which was designed by nature to help us digest our foods properly. Remember that our digestion actually begins with the secretion of enzymes in our saliva at the smell and appearance of food. In Thailand, where mangoes grow in abundance, this fruit's fragrance is intoxicating. I know that personally, because I spent time in Thailand years ago, and still go there once a year to teach at the anti-aging hospital in Bangkok. Yet I'd never know about that wonderful smell from the mangoes sitting in a store in Seattle. Eating organic and local isn't trendy. It's better for you.

The Best and Worst Nonorganic Foods

I understand that not everyone chooses to (or can) go completely organic. If you can't or won't, you can pick and choose the nonorganic fruits and vegetables that are least damaging. Of course, the more organic foods you eat, the lower the amount of pesticides and chemicals your liver has to deal with.

The Environmental Working Group, a national nonprofit organization that conducts research on the chemicals and additives in products we use and consume, compiles a list of the most contaminated nonorganic fruits and vegetables. "The Dirty Dozen," is currently titled "The Dirty Dozen Plus" because more than twelve are listed. "The Clean Fifteen," is a list of the least contaminated nonorganic fruits and vegetables.

THE DIRTY DOZEN PLUS	THE CLEAN FIFTEEN
Apples	Asparagus
Bell peppers	Avocados
Celery	Cabbage
Cherry tomatoes	Cantaloupes
Cucumbers	Corn
Grapes	Eggplants
Hot chili peppers	Grapefruits
Kale/collard greens	Kiwis
Nectarines, imported	Mangoes
Peaches	Mushrooms
Potatoes	Onions
Spinach	Papayas
Strawberries	Peas, frozen
Summer squash	Pineapples
	Sweet potatoes

Why are some fruits and vegetables more susceptible to contamination than others? Foods like strawberries seem to absorb pesticides more easily. It's almost as if they attract and become supersaturated with chemicals. Apples have a similar susceptibility. Of course, we also eat the skin of apples, which has a waxy film that should be cleaned off. But how many of us wash our fruits and vegetables with soap and water? I do. If you don't (which would place you in the majority), you can do one of two things: Vigorously wash produce with a sponge or a scrub brush. Follow by rinsing off the soap completely. Or you can soak fruits and vegetables in a sink full of water using the produce cleaning liquid available in grocery stores. You'll be amazed at the amount of yucky residue that's left in the sink. Or just use vinegar (one part vinegar to three parts water). The acidic blend kills all the bacteria. The solution also kills E. coli, including the strain E. coli 0157:H7, which can be lethal.

There's another reason to wash produce. Did you know that washing berries, including strawberries, with a vinegar solution prevents them from molding within a few days of purchase? Have you ever bought raspberries and found that, twenty-four hours later, they were bad? Just be sure to rinse your berries very well and let them air-dry before storing them in a container.

Grow Your Own Sprouts

According to the Centers for Disease Control (CDC), forty-eight million Americans—one in six—get sick from foodborne illnesses annually. Outbreaks caused by both imported and domestic fruits and vegetables have increased in recent years, and have occurred after eating produce such as sprouts, lettuce, apples, cantaloupes, and other produce. E. coli 0157:H7 particularly shows up in sprouts. Because sprouts do not handle vinegar washing well, I recommend growing your own. They are easy and inexpensive to grow, look pretty, and you will use them more when they're always available.

Sprouts are everyday seeds, beans, or grains that have been soaked, rinsed, and allowed to germinate (sprout) for a few days before you eat them. The easiest options are alfalfa, mustard, radish, and clover. You can also use legumes: lentils, mung beans, garbanzos, and green peas are all good choices to start with.

Select your seeds based on taste preference. If you like the small sprouts like alfalfa, which are often used in salads, sandwiches, and spring rolls, start with seeds. If you prefer beans, lentils, and peas, which are wonderful in stir-fry, salad, or soup, use those. Sprouted legumes require much less cooking time than dried legumes and are also more tender.

The legumes should be "seed quality," which is generally recommended for sprouting, as compared with "food quality," which is intended for cooking. These can be found in most health-food stores, often in the bulk bins, or in specialty shops, and are also available online. My favorite online source is www.sproutpeople .org. Once you have your seeds in hand, store them in airtight containers until you're ready to use them. Glass jars work well for this purpose.

Setting Up

Growing Supplies
- ✧ Widemouthed Mason jars sized from 1 quart to 1 gallon are recommended, depending on the amount of seed you want.
- ✧ Cheesecloth
- ✧ Rubber bands, or you can use the outer part of the top of the Mason jar to screw over the screen.
- ✧ Dish rack or flat, shallow containers for the jars to drain into.

During the germination process, sprouts prefer a dark, temperate (60° to 85°F) location, away from drafts and direct heat. An empty cabinet, box, or dish rack covered with cloth will work well.

Sprouting

1. Measure out your seeds or beans; 1 ounce of seed yields about 1 cup of sprouts, so ¼ cup (for a 2-cup yield) is a good starting point for small seed sprouts. Soaked beans and legumes expand to approximately double the amount of dried ones. Place seeds in a mesh strainer or in your sprouting jar and rinse in warm (80°F) water.

2. If you used a strainer for rinsing, pour seeds or legumes into your Mason jar. Fill ¾ with water, cap with cheesecloth and lid or rubber band, and let soak overnight (if prepared in the evening) or for the following times:

 ✧ Small seeds: 3–8 hours
 ✧ Larger seeds or legumes: 8–16 hours
 ✧ Grains: 16–20 hours

3. Drain the water and rinse the seeds thoroughly. Rinse them two to three times daily.

4. After each rinse, place the jar upside down and tilted at a 45-degree angle in the warm, dark germination spot you've selected. Keep your growing sprouts damp but not soaking. A warm dark location will make them sprout faster.

5. Let the sprouts germinate for the suggested number of days. See the germination chart at drtami.com.

6. Once seeds have sprouted, place the jar in strong, indirect sunlight for two to three days to develop some nutrient-rich chlorophyll. (Do not do this for legumes.)

7. When the jar is full and the sprouts or legumes are ready for use, store in an airtight container (a capped sprouting jar is fine) in the refrigerator. Note: Be sure sprouts have drained for at least five

hours before storing; too much moisture can cause spoilage. If you'd prefer to see the video of these instructions, see drtami.com under Recipes.

What You Need to Know About GMOs

Introduced in the United States twenty years ago, GMOs (genetically modified organisms) have become a huge factor in the American diet today. Although most of us are unaware of it, GMOs are now used to make the ingredients of roughly 80 percent of packaged foods, according to a front-page article in the *Wall Street Journal* in August 2014. Over 90 percent of corn, soybeans, and sugar beets are GMOs.

Why is this important? The genetic makeup of GMO foods has been manipulated to create or improve positive characteristics, such as resistance to weeds, or to enhance vitamins and nutrients. The problem is we don't know the long-term damage GMOs may cause to the environment—and to us. I recently spoke with Jeffrey M. Smith, bestselling author and authority on GMOs, and a top advocate for non-GMO nutrition. Smith notes that early studies show increases in tumors, decreases in hormones and fertility, and other serious health problems. Although the studies were done on rats, early medical research is usually on rats, not humans.

The United States has embraced GMO foods on the premise that GMOs haven't proven to be dangerous. In contrast, Europe, for the most part, has banned GMOs saying GMOs haven't proven to be safe. Last year, the United States granted Monsanto (which makes GMOs) a waiver that exempts it from all possible lawsuits due to future harm by GMOs. No suing for damages.

Most important, you usually don't know if you're eating GMO

foods or not because these foods are not required to be labeled. Vermont is the first state to require GMO labeling (beginning in 2016).

How can you protect yourself and your family and remove GMOs from your diet? Jeffrey Smith advises, "One of the best things you can do is eat organic. 'Certified organic' means no GMO seeds or pesticides have been used, but they haven't been tested. It's possible there may be some cross-contamination because these chemicals can drift into air, rain, and water."

You can also look for foods labeled Non GMO, indicating they've been tested and found to have no genetically modified organisms. So if you're really worried, the label should read Non GMO and certified organic. There aren't many products that carry that label yet. In addition to the crops already mentioned, alfalfa, sorghum, and currently, wheat are genetically modified, according to Jeffrey Smith. You need to know the facts, so you can choose your level of effort and comfort.

The Toxins in Everything Else

Every single part of your life is either harming you or optimizing you. There is no middle ground. Take xenoestrogens, for example. These are compounds with estrogen-like activity. However, it's bad estrogen activity that's associated with the increased risk of cancer. The problem is that xenoestrogens are everywhere. You get up in the morning and brush your teeth. But have you ever read your toothpaste label? If you swallow any paste, you're supposed to call poison control. Take a look in your shower. The soap, shampoo, and conditioners on the shelf all contain parabens, chemical preservatives that extend their shelf life. Parabens are also xenoestrogens. The towel you use to dry yourself contains residue from laundry detergent and fabric softeners that have xenoestrogens. And you put that residue in contact with the largest organ of your body—your skin.

If you drink nonorganic coffee, you ingest pesticides, which are xenoestrogens. And decaf has its own problems. Often it's decaffeinated with methylene chloride, which the federal Occupational Safety and Health Administration (OSHA) calls a potent human carcinogen. The amount left on coffee beans during this process is said to be minimal, but I encourage you to avoid toxins whenever possible. The Swiss decaffeination process uses water and is thought to be the safest way to decaffeinate coffee.

Finally, let's say the boss hands you a bonus, and you celebrate by buying a new car. You swing open the door, slide in, and inhale the satisfying "new-car smell"—which is produced by one of the most dangerous xenoestrogens, phthalates. Phthalates make plastics more flexible and harder to break.

Almost all hair conditioners are harmful. It took me twenty-five minutes at a department store to find one suitable for my daughter, who is only eight years old and has crazy-curly hair. I almost gave up on finding one without chemicals that act like xenoestrogens and disrupt hormones. I can't expose her to fake chemical estrogen. We think such chemicals, plus the hormones in chickens, milk, and meat, may have something to do with the fact that puberty is developing earlier and earlier in girls in this country.

Antiperspirants/deodorants are another issue. First, let me explain the difference between the two. Antiperspirants attempt to stop you from perspiring; deodorants attempt to ensure that your perspiration doesn't smell bad. Antiperspirants are much worse, because they contain aluminum. Studies to determine whether aluminum might cause Alzheimer's disease were not well done (and used rabbits). Controversy continues about a possible connection between the two. Nevertheless, we do know that aluminum is not good for the brain (and tends to want to go to the brain). Aluminum also forms a temporary sweat-duct plug. What's wrong with that? Remember, sweating is the body's way of expelling toxins. Your body retains those toxins if you don't perspire.

Sweat itself doesn't smell. It's the combination of perspiration, hormones, bacteria, and other substances that causes body odor. Deodorants are preferable to antiperspirants because they allow us to sweat, yet also mask the odor. My personal favorite deodorant is Arm & Hammer Essentials, which does not contain aluminum, is paraben-free, and uses natural deodorizers. There are other brands of natural deodorant, such as Tom's of Maine, that do not contain aluminum.

The deodorant issue is critically important for girls, because they start to experience body odor between the ages of nine and eleven. Body odor is one of the very first signs of puberty. A period can be expected within a year or two. And what are you going to give a nine-year-old that won't disrupt her hormones? Definitely a deodorant, not an antiperspirant. There are so many things in your life that you can't control, but this is something that you can.

Although cosmetics and toiletries free of preservatives and other potentially harmful substances can be hard to find, they are available. Fortunately, you just have to do the research once. After you find the shampoo that you feel comfortable with, you can head directly to that brand. But the first time you're going to have to read labels. My online shopping cart on drtami.com can help. I list foods, personal and health-care products, and other items that carry my stamp of approval. Finding the best, most affordable, and healthiest options can be time-consuming. I've done the research for you.

Talking to the Right Physician

Another issue you can do something about is hiring or firing your doctor. Your own research on the Internet may or may not be appropriate for a complex system like the body—plus, lots of misinformation appears online. Even absolutely correct information may not be right for your individual case. Therefore, you need the help of your doctor to interpret research and separate fact from fiction. You also want a health-care provider who is willing to work with you—and, ideally, one who has received extra training in integrative or anti-aging medicine. Why? Because all medical training is disease-oriented. I went to medical school for a very long time, and was never taught about the alternative ways in which nutrition, supplements, and lifestyle changes can prevent and treat conditions.

If your physician is an ob-gyn or an endocrinologist who has studied hormones, this does not guarantee that she/he knows or understands natural ways of working with your body to balance and boost the symphony of hormones. The education of such specialists has been focused entirely on disease and on pharmaceutical and surgical solutions to health issues. You need to find someone who has added to her/his education by learning alternative ways of treating the body. I regularly refer my patients to a gynecologist to get an ultrasound to investigate a uterine fibroid and a surgical solution to take it out. What I have found, however, is that gynecologists often do not go on to investigate why the fibroid grew and how to make sure another one doesn't grow back. That's where natural medicine comes in.

An option is to go to a physician who is educated above and beyond traditional medicine. You can find a huge list on the website of the American Academy of Anti-Aging Medicine, http://www.a4m .com. The MDs listed have received a fellowship or board certification in anti-aging medicine.

Many naturopaths, health practitioners who are not MDs but

focus exclusively on natural medicine, are well versed in prescribing bioidentical hormones. However, some naturopaths believe that bioidentical hormones are unnecessary and that the body can produce all that is needed. Unfortunately, that is not always the case.

Other naturopaths are open to prescriptions. Sometimes insurance companies will pay for a naturopath. It's a personal choice. But if you see a naturopath, make sure the person is educated in hormones. Not all naturopaths are.

Some patients tell me that their primary-care physician or gynecologist freaks out when she/he hears that I've prescribed bioidentical hormones. These doctors say, "There's no proof that this works, and I won't see you if you continue to do this." I encourage you to find a physician who is supportive and excited that you're getting the help you need—a doctor who responds, "Ha, I never had any training in this stuff. Just tell Dr. Smith to send me her notes so I know what's going on."

Find someone who knows that it takes a team to support a patient's health. One doctor became angry with a patient of mine because she was seeing another doctor for issues that he felt he could take care of. She told him, "If I had a bone problem, you'd send me to a bone surgeon. If I had a heart problem, you'd send me to a cardiologist. Well, I have a hormone problem, and I'm seeing an MD who specializes in hormones. You should be happy."

I remember examining a forty-four-year-old man whose PSA (prostate-specific antigen, the protein produced by prostate cells) was below 4 (which is considered normal), yet it had risen twice in less than a year. I told him, "I don't know why, but this bugs me. I really want you to see a urologist." He did, and was given a diagnosis of prostate cancer. The urologist asked, "Why did your doctor send you? Your PSA was normal. She may have saved your life." I had told the patient, "I don't know what to do about this, so I'll send you to someone who might."

Another patient, who is taking bioidentical hormones, has multiple sclerosis (MS). I don't know how all these hormones interact with MS. I said to her, "Tell me who follows you for your MS, because I must consult with him/her." Doctors are expected to be the experts, and it's hard for some to admit, "I don't know."

These two patients are doing well. The woman who told her doctor that he should be happy she's seeing a hormone specialist took bioidentical hormones for only a short while. She began sleeping better for the first time in years, and she was weaned off hormones because she didn't want to stay on them forever. She's handling her problems with nutritional supplements and lifestyle changes, and she feels great. However, women who do want to stay on hormones can do so safely with low, customized doses of bioidenticals that are appropriate for their individual health status.

Understanding Customized Medicine

Today, we practice mainly "chemical medicine," even in my anti-aging specialty, where we give hormones and nutritional supplements. We look for problems in the chemistry of the body by taking blood and urine tests. And we treat the problems with medications, such as calcium and serotonin, that alter the chemistry. But we're not just chemistry. We're also energetic. The heart has electrical activity, and we diagnose cardiac problems with an electrocardiogram (EKG). We give you a pill (aka a chemical) for treatment, but it's an electrical issue. How do you restart a heart? You shock it with electricity. Our brain is also electrical. There's so much in our world that is electrical surrounding us. And we really have no idea how these things affect our health and well-being. We're constantly bombarded with electrical frequencies and energetic interference. We sit in front of computers all day and TV all night. We hold cell phones literally up to our ear and brain. We do know there's been a big increase in brain cancer recently. There's no proof at this time that it's related to cell-phone use, but it's something to think about. When I was in medical school, brain cancer was considered a rare cancer.

We physicians look at a computer and at test results. How people feel is largely ignored, even though it affects their well-being. Learning how a patient feels requires that your doctor listen to you. If you're not feeling "heard" as a patient, you need to speak up.

I often say, "I'd love to be able to read your mind, but I cannot. I need you to tell me everything you feel and what's bothering you, whether or not you think I'll agree—because I actually have plans A through W that I can create for you. If one doesn't work, we'll try something else." This is a very different model from just seeing a doctor who tells you what to do, or makes you feel ashamed if you question his/her directions or ask about alternatives. Many women are told to take an antidepressant they don't want. They never return, because it's too uncomfortable to say no to the doctor, who will proceed to criticize them.

Doctor-patient communication is much better than it used to be. But lack of understanding still happens, especially because physicians have only fifteen minutes for each visit and don't have the luxury of explaining why and what the alternatives could be and what the lifestyle options are.

You also want to find a health provider who (1) understands optimal hormonal ranges, (2) looks at optimal ranges but treats *you* (not your test results), (3) customizes bioidentical hormones if you need them and uses a Pharmacy Compounding Accreditation Board (PCAB) pharmacy, (4) listens to you, and (5) doesn't hesitate to say, "I don't know." (6) Your doctor should also have an extensive intake form. He/she should want to know about your family history and medical history, because nothing works in isolation. Everything we do affects everything else.

Tests You Can Discuss with Your Doctor

Every single hormone and nutrient has an optimal blood-test range, and certain blood tests can uncover deficiencies that you can talk about with your physician. I didn't learn about optimal ranges in hormones, vitamins, and minerals in laboratory testing in medical school. I learned about this during years of additional postgraduate training. The reference ranges used by the medical establishment are disease ranges. That means the bare minimum to avoid disease.

For example, the reference range for vitamin D is 30 or 32–100, depending on the laboratory. The optimal range is 60–100, as shown in the chart on pages 248–249 The medical-establishment reference range for cortisol is 2.9µg/dL-25. The optimal range is 12–15.

The vitamin C range is the minimum to avoid getting scurvy. You and your doctor need to think way beyond disease ranges in evaluating the range your hormones should be in order for you to live vibrantly and prevent the diseases and conditions associated with aging. These optimal ranges have been well studied and used in integrative medicine for more than thirty years to prove they are safe.

I have patients who are not in the optimal ranges but feel great. Their hot flashes, night sweats, and brain fog have stopped. They feel energized. Their body forgot to read the textbook. Their optimal range is different. You want somebody who uses customized medicine—not "Take this one prescription for Prozac. One size fits all."

Many lab reference ranges are very wide. For example, a "normal" thyroid range runs from the floor to the ceiling. But what if you were in the upper third of the reference range in your twenties, and now, in your forties and fifties, you're in the lower third? You're still "normal," but that's a huge drop that affects how your body functions and feels. We don't know what our own optimal ranges are.

We're not testing for it in our young people. Every single hormone and nutrient has an optimal range.

Everybody says, "Oh, my doctor did a liver-function test (LFT) and I'm fine." This tests to see if your liver is so injured that it's leaching enzymes into the bloodstream. The LFT tells us if your liver is sick, but not if the liver is working optimally. You could be on the

---

IDEAL FEMALE BLOOD LEVELS

If your own nonprescription boosting and balancing of hormones isn't sufficient, you really need to be monitored by a health-care professional who can create the perfect doses of bioidenticals for your individual case. She/he will look at results of your lab tests below for safety, and factor in how you feel, to calibrate the hormones that will correct your symptoms.

The fact is, your blood pressure, heart rate, and other medical tests may be normal, and you still may not feel well. It isn't all in your head. It's real. Below are blood tests that I consider to be essential, plus the optimal range for each.

- ❖ Testosterone (Free): 8 pg/ml or 28 pmol/L
- ❖ Testosterone (Total): 35 ng/dl or 1.2 mmol/L
- ❖ Estradiol: 60–100 pg/ml
- ❖ Progesterone: 2–8 ng/ml
- ❖ DHEA-S: 175–330 ug/dL
- ❖ Cortisol (Free): 20 ng/ml or 55 mmol/L
- ❖ Cortisol (Total): 180 ng/ml or 550 mmol/L
- ❖ Transcortin[1]: 30 mg/L
- ❖ T3 (Free): 2.5–3.4 ng/dl or 3.9–5.2 pmol/L
- ❖ T4 (Free): 1.3–1.8 ng/dl or 16.7–23.2 pmol/L
- ❖ TSH[2]: 0.4–1.0 ulU/mL

---

verge of big problems and it wouldn't show up. The LFT is a great test for assessing diseases of the liver, but it has nothing to do with optimal functioning.

One of the blood tests I suggest you discuss with your doctor is an intracellular test of sufficiencies in vitamins and minerals. I also suggest vitamin D 25-0H hydroxy. A patient came to me last week

- ❖ IGF-1[3]: 250–300 mcg/L or 28–40
- ❖ SHBG[4]: 65 any day
- ❖ Ferritin[5]: 80–100
- ❖ CRP[6]: low risk <1.0 mg/L; average risk 1.0–3.0 mg/L; high risk >3.0 mg/L
- ❖ Fasting insulin test: 2–5
- ❖ Vitamin D 25-OH: 60–100 ng/ml
- ❖ Full cholesterol panel once a year

---

[1] Globulin that binds cortisol, rendering it inactive

[2] Thyroid test

[3] Best blood test for levels of human growth hormone

[4] Sex hormone-binding globulin. Controls amount of free testosterone.

[5] Tests amount of iron in body

[6] Test for inflammation in body

Note: Through the process of medical metabolism, hormones can be converted into other hormones. For example, estradiol can turn into 2-hydroxyestrone or 4- or 16-hydroxyestrone. Each has a different impact on your health. You don't know if the conversion of estradiol to these metabolites has been completed. The best place to test these "end metabolites" is at the end. And that means a urine test. Ask your doctor to check your urine at the end of testing to be sure your hormones are safe. Physicians should look at the whole person. All of us change over time.

whose primary-care doctor wanted her to stop taking her vitamin D because her levels were "high." She brought in the results of the test he had taken, and the test did show an elevated level. But a few days later we got the Vitamin D 25-0H test, which is considered *the* test to use, and it showed her levels to be low normal, not high. She had originally gotten the least expensive and the least helpful vitamin D test. Her doctor was going to give her bad advice based on a lab test that didn't give her any physiological information. It's like saying how much food is in the grocery store. That has nothing to do with how much food you have on your table.

Where to Find Labs on Your Own

If you wish to order your own lab tests at any time, here are some options:

1. Vitality Medispa and Medical Clinic. At my clinic, we sell a blood spot finger-prick test that gives results equal in accuracy to a blood-serum test. The test kit is shipped to you, and the shipping label to send to the lab is included.
2. Genova Diagnostics, http://www.gdx.net. They have great hormone evaluations.
3. Mymedialab.com. Offers a variety of blood tests.
4. Life Extension. You can order a comprehensive hormone blood test.

For further reading, see the resources section on page 265.

Vitamins and Herbs—Caveat

I think we take way too many vitamins. It's not that they're bad, but they're sometimes unnecessary and a waste of money. Not all vitamin supplements are created equal. They're not monitored by the FDA, because they aren't foods and aren't drugs. A vitamin labeled 250 mg of vitamin C might or might not have 250 mg. It could have 5 mg—and it's perfectly legal. We rely on the honesty and accuracy of the manufacturer to ensure that each and every tablet contains what is on the label, and what is in the pill is listed on the label. A study published in 2013 in *JAMA Internal Medicine* revealed that researchers who tested vitamin D pills sold in stores found that they contained 9 percent to 40 percent of the doses listed on the labels. In addition, one-third of multivitamins tested by ConsumerLabs in 2009 was contaminated or contained significantly more or less of some ingredients than the labels claimed. The good news is that there are some vitamin companies that have volunteered to hold themselves accountable. The way you can be sure that the supplement you are buying is accurately labeled is to look for the following:

1. GMP (Good Manufacturing Practices) stamp. GMP regulations, established by the Food and Drug Administration (FDA), tells you the manufacturing conditions for drugs and supplements in the United States meet minimum standards.
2. USP (United States Pharmacopoeia) Verified Mark. This indicates that a supplement has been voluntarily submitted to the USP by the manufacturer and has met the criteria of performance, consistency, and current FDA good manufacturing practices.
3. NSF (National Sanitation Foundation). This is an independent agency that tests and certifies products.

The Rest of the Supplement Story

Buying vitamins and minerals with the seals of approval listed above on the label is only part of the story. My good friends and colleagues Dr. Jayson and Mira Calton, who are experts in micronutrients, say that we should look for the ABCs as well:

A: Absorbable.

A good start is to make sure the vitamin pills dissolve in a glass of water, but further studies should show that your cells absorb these vital nutrients to ensure that you're not flushing them down the toilet, literally.

I did a piece on vitamin absorption as the health and beauty expert for our local TV news. The segment started out by putting certain top-selling multivitamins in a glass of water to see whether they would dissolve. Many hours later, some of the vitamins still hadn't started to dissolve. This is important, because the pill will remain in your stomach indefinitely. It's going to transfer through your system, and before your body can absorb it, it has to dissolve. The most amazing pill in the world won't help you if you can't break it down and absorb it.

Realize, too, that liquids are more easily dissolved than capsules, and capsules are more easily absorbed than tablets. For example, Nutreince multivitamin (Calton Nutrition) dissolves easily in water and is easier to absorb. It comes in great flavors and encourages you to drink water.

I changed a patient's vitamin D to Nutreince as an experiment to see if I could increase her absorption, because she's a young woman with osteopenia. Her blood tests showed that she also had low levels of calcium and vitamin D. She had been taking pharmaceutical-grade vitamins approved by me for almost a year, yet she still had absorption problems. At her three-month follow-up, her vitamin D and calcium levels were up, despite the fact that she was taking "less." She had switched to taking Nutreince in her water daily, and her blood tests proved that her absorption had increased.

B: Beneficial quantities and forms.

We want optimal levels of micronutrients, not minimum levels. The RDA recommended daily allowances represent the minimal amount of a nutrient necessary to prevent disease. For example, vitamin C deficiency causes scurvy. Scurvy presents with bleeding gums, spots on the skin, and profound fatigue, and is rarely seen today. Scurvy was first described by Hippocrates and was prevalent in the Age of Discovery, when sailing voyages lasted longer than fresh fruit and vegetables on the ship. The Reference Daily Intake (RDI) is a much better measurement, and is described as the amount of micronutrients needed for 97 percent to 98 percent of healthy individuals. This is an important reminder that we all need more micronutrient help when we aren't feeling well or when we're fighting diseases.

C: Competition.
Today, forty-two different micronutrient competitions have been discovered that can prevent the absorption of your supplements. For example, zinc competes with copper. If you take zinc without also taking copper, you will create a copper deficiency.

S: Synergies.
Synergies are vitamins and minerals that work together and aid absorption. Vitamins and minerals require the same delicate balance as the hormone orchestra.

When I practiced medicine in a hospital setting, we gave our anemic patients their iron supplements with applesauce, because iron is best absorbed in an acidic environment. We can help the body absorb fat-soluble vitamins by taking them when we consume fat. The fat-soluble vitamins are A, D, E, and K. So the omega-3 fatty acids found in fish oil are great to take with your vitamin D.

◆　◆　◆

You may not be getting what you think you're buying in herbal remedies, either. A study of herbal-product integrity and authenticity published in the journal *BMC Medicine* in 2013 found poor quality in most of the forty-four herbal products and fifty leaf samples from forty-two herbal species tested. Of the products tested, 59 percent contained DNA bar codes from plant species not listed on the labels. Many also contained contaminants (some of which posed serious health risks) and/or fillers unlisted on the label. The World Health Organization considers the adulteration of herbal products a threat to consumer safety.

Be the CEO of Your Own Health

I just received a note from a new patient, the mother of two toddlers. It reads:

"I wanted to report that I feel *amazing* after one week. I started treatment with you on July 22nd, and by the 29th I had more energy and did more projects around the house in a forty-eight-hour period than I had in the past six months combined. I feel that I have been lifted out of a fog. I'm more motivated, more even in my mood, more apt to just get up and do things as opposed to feeling like a slug. My weight is steadily declining—up to a pound a day almost. My husband is very excited about my new breath of fresh air. It's exactly what I needed and I feel a gazillion times better. You are incredible. I never want to go back to the way I was living. I feel like I was under a rock for months. Eternally grateful, Laura."

Laura went to the doctor because she felt tired all the time—and was told that nothing was wrong. She assumed that was the way it is for a stay-at-home mom with young children. However, Laura was only in her thirties, and her mom, who is a patient of mine, said, "You have to go to Dr. Tami and see if there's something more."

I ran a series of tests on Laura, and uncovered a progesterone deficiency and a sluggish thyroid. We also discussed nutrition. She told me, "We eat pretty well. I stay home, so I have time to shop and cook." When we talked about the specifics of her diet, it became apparent that she was not eating for energy.

I prescribed my thirty-day program. Now she feels that she got her life back. Laura was not sick, but, like many women, she believed she was in a slow decline and that feeling less than her best was "normal." Women constantly hear, "What do you expect? You have small children." "What do you expect? You're in menopause." "What do you expect? You work and have kids." We're always told there's a reason that we don't feel fabulous. But it's not the true reason.

Yes, our years of perimenopause and menopause are associated with more significant physical changes than at any other time in our lives except puberty. But these shifts needn't drain the life out of us. They can be addressed. I hope you will stick to the changes you've made, and that you'll refer to this book periodically, whenever you have questions or concerns.

I also challenge you to make an appointment with your iPhone every day for optimal health. Everything that is important finds its way onto our calendars. Women often feel more than a little guilty about things that they do not do. Turn this guilt into an advantage. I used to have a meditation reminder on my phone calendar, and I would often hear the alarm and say, "Yes, I will get to that in a minute." The minutes, then the day, then the week went by with no meditation. I now have a new reminder. My meditation alarm reads, "Time for meditation so I will be healthy and strong enough to see my girls graduate, marry, and have their own children." That is a hard one to say "I don't have time" for! We women make appointments for our children, the dog, our own parents, our job—and not for ourselves. If not now, when?

Let your grocery store be your pharmacy. Let meditation be your tranquilizer. And make your decisions count every day.

Acknowledgments

This book would not have been possible without the love and support of my best friend and love of my life, my husband, Rocco. Many hours he has listened (and still listens) to my musings about medicine and how I might improve how it is practiced. I also owe a special love-filled thank-you to my parents, who have supported me from ballet career to medicine and motherhood. A special thank-you to my mother-in-law, Cosimina, whose amazing recipes Rocco and I were able to take and make Hormone Healthy.

I would also like to acknowledge my agent, Celeste Fine, who believed in me and was instrumental in helping flesh out my initial ideas to make the work I do with patients every day something that could bless more than one patient at a time. I also want to acknowledge the people at Atria for their support in helping get this important information into print.

I want to say a heartfelt thank-you to Florence Isaacs, a truly gifted wordsmith. She was able to take all my words, research, knowledge, and humor and craft them into a flowing piece that is filled with both inspiration and life-changing information. She is an artist.

I am grateful for my amazing team at my clinic. My operations manager, Lindsey Monteith, provided tremendous support during this process.

Thank you to my wonderful photographers, Stacie and Darrell Peterson.

I also want to say a special thank-you to Daniel Amen, who encouraged me to write this book and helped me learn the steps and introduced me to many of the people that have made this possible. I am grateful to Jeff Hays, Jayson and Mira Calton, Leanne Ely, Pedram Shojai, Bill Harris, and JJ Virgin for their guidance and insights.

And finally, thank you to my patients for allowing me into your lives to help fill you with more energy, life, and vitality. I love you all.

Notes

CHAPTER 1

University of Rochester Medical Center, "Cognitive difficulties associated with menopause described," *Science Daily* (January 2013).

"Early Surgical Menopause Is Associated with a Spectrum of Cognitive Decline," 65th Annual Meeting, American Academy of Neurology (March 16–23, 2013).

Susan Rako, "Testosterone Supplemental Therapy after Hysterectomy with or without Concomitant Oophorectomy: Estrogen Alone Is Not Enough," *Journal of Women's Health & Gender-Based Medicine* (October 2000): 9 (8); 917–923.

CHAPTER 2

K. K. Miller, B. M. K. Biller, C. Beauregard, et al., "Effects of Testosterone Replacement in Androgen-Deficient Women with Hypopituitarism: A Randomized, Double-Blind, Placebo-Controlled Study," *Journal of Clinical Endocrinology & Metabolism* vol. 91, no. 5 (2006): 1683–1690.

C. Wang, R. S. Swerdloff, A. Iranmanesh, et al., "Effects of transdermal testosterone gel on bone turnover markets and bone mineral density in hypogonadal men," *Clinical Endocrinology* (2001): 54 (6): 739–50, http://www/ncbi.nlm.nih.gov/pubmed/11422108.

Nicole Carter and Mohamed Kabbaj, "Extracellular Signal-Regulated Kinase 2 Signaling in the Hippocampal Dentate Gyrus Mediates the Antidepressant Effects of Testosterone," *Biological Psychiatry* (2012): 71 (7): 642–65, doi:10.1016.

F. A. Zarrouf, S. Artz, et al., "Testosterone and depression: systematic review and meta-analysis," *Journal of Psychiatric Practice* (2009): 15 (4): 289–305.

Louann Brizendine, MD, "Managing menopause-related depression and low libido," *The Journal of Family Practice* vol. 16, no. 8 (2004).

U. D. Rohr, "The impact of testosterone imbalance on depression and women's health," *Maturitas* (April 15, 2002): 41 suppl. 1:S25–46.

Scott D. Moffat and Susan M. Resnick, "Long term measures of free testosterone predict regional cerebral blood flow patterns in elderly men," *Neurobiology of Aging* vol. 28 (6): 914–920 (2007).

Sonia L. Davison, Robin J. Bell, Maria Gavrilescu, et al., "Testosterone improves verbal learning and memory in postmenopausal women, results from a pilot study," *Maturitas* vol. 70, no. 3 (November 2011): 307–311.

G. M. Rosano et al., "Testosterone therapy in women with chronic heart failure: A pilot double-blind, randomized, placebo-controlled study," *Journal of the American College of Cardiology* (2010): 12; 56 (16):1310–6.

Shalender Bhasin, Glenn R. Cunningham, et al., "Testosterone Therapy in Adult Men with Androgen Deficiency Syndromes: An Endocrine Society Clinical Practice Guideline" (2006), *The Journal of Clinical Endocrinology & Metabolism,* doi: http://dx.doi.org/10.1210/jc.2005-2847.

Gail A. Laughlin, Vivian Goodell, et al., "Extremes of Endogenous Testosterone Are Associated with Increased Risk of Incident Coronary Events in Older Women," *Journal of Clinical Endocrinology and Metabolism* (2010), doi:http//dx.doi.org/10–1210/ju.2009–1693.

Caroline Sievers, Jens Klotsche, Lars Pieper, et al., "Low testosterone levels predict all-cause mortality and cardiovascular events in women: A prospective cohort study in German primary care patients," *European Journal of Endocrinology* (October 1, 2010): 163, 699–708.

Susan R. Davis, MBBS, FRACP, PhD and Sonia L. Davidson, MBBS, FRACP, PhD, "Current perspectives on testosterone therapy for women," *Menopausal Medicine* vol. 20, no. 2 (May 2012).

Erik Debing, Els Peeters, William Duquet, et al., "Endogenous sex hormone levels in postmenopausal women undergoing carotid artery endarterectomy," *European Journal of Endocrinology* (2007): 156 (6): 687–693, doi:10.1530/EJE-06-0702.

J. L. Shifren, The role of androgens in female sexual dysfunction, *Mayo Clinic Proceedings*, 79 suppl. (2004): S19–24.

Jan L. Shifren, MD; Glenn D. Braunstein, MD; et al., "Transdermal Testosterone Treatment in Women with Impaired Sexual Function after Oophorectomy," *New England Journal of Medicine* (2000): 343: 682–8.

Marie Hofling, MD; Angelica Linden Hirschberg, MD, PhD; Lambert Skoog, MD, PhD; et al., "Testosterone inhibits estrogen/progestogen-induced breast cell proliferation in postmenopausal women," *Menopause* vol. 14, no. 2 (2007): 183–89.

Federation of American Society for Experimental Biology. *The FASEB Journal* (September 2000). http://journals.Iww.com/menopausejournal /Abstract/2007/14020/Testosterone_inhibits_estrogen_progestogen _induced.5.aspx.

Susan R. Davis, MBBS, FRACP, PhD and Sonia L. Davidson, MBBS, FRACP, PhD, "Current perspectives on testosterone therapy for women," *Menopausal Medicine*, vol. 20, no. 2 (May 2012).

CHAPTER 3

A. S. Prasad et al., "Mineral supplements increase testosterone levels," *Nutrition* (1996), 12.5:344–48.

Lara E. Laugsand, Linn B. Strand, et al., "Insomnia and the risk of incident heart failure: a population study," *European Heart Journal* (2013), doi.10.1093/eurheartj/eht019.

Sanjay R. Patel, Atul Malhotra, et al., "Association Between Reduced Sleep and Weight Gain in Women," *American Journal of Epidemiology* (2006): 164 (10): 947–954.

Daniel F. Kripke, Robert D. Langer, Lawrence E. Kline, "Hypnotics' association with mortality or cancer: a matched cohort study," *BMJ Open* 2012; 2:e000850, doi:10.1136/bmjopen-2012-00850.

Amnon Brzezinski, Mark G. Vangel, et al., "Effects of exogenous melatonin on sleep: a meta-analysis," *Sleep Medicine Reviews* (2005): 9, 41–50.

Tierney A. Lorenz, MA, and Cindy M. Meston, "Acute Exercise Improves Physical Sexual Arousal in Women Taking Antidepressants," *Annals of Behavioral Medicine* (June 2012): 43 (3): 352–361, doi: 10.1007/s 12 160-011-9338-1.

D. M. Lithgow and W. M. Politzer, "Vitamin A in the treatment of menorrhagia," *South African Medical Journal* (1977): 51: 191–193.

Mindy S. Kurzer, PhD et al., "Effects of Aerobic Exercise on Estrogen Metabolism in Healthy Premenopausal Women," *Cancer Epidemiology, Biomarkers & Prevention* (2013): 22; 756.

CHAPTER 4

C. R. MacLean, K. G. Walton, S. R. Wenneberg, et al., "Effects of the Transcendental Meditation Program on adaptive mechanisms: changes in hormone levels and responses to stress after 4 months of practice," *Psychoneuroendocrinology* (May 1997): 22 (4): 277–95.

Michael Mrazek et al., "Mindfulness Training Improves Working Memory Capacity and GRE Performance While Reducing Mind Wandering," *Psychological Science* (2013).

Joel W. Hughes, PhD; David M. Fresco, PhD; Rodney Myerscough, PhD; et al., "Randomized Controlled Trial of Mindfulness-Based Stress Reduction for Prehypertension," *Psychosomatic Medicine* vol. 75, no. 8 (2013): 721–728.

CHAPTER 6

Gemma Flores-Mateo, David Rojas-Rueda, Josep Basoa, et al., "Nutritional intake and adiposity: meta-analysis of clinical trials," *American Journal of Clinical Nutrition* (2013): ajcn.031484.

Ying Bao, MD, ScD; Jiali Han, PhD; et al., "Association of Nut Consumption with Total and Cause-Specific Mortality," *New England Journal of Medicine* (2013): 369: 2001–2011.

M. Garaulet, P. Gómez-Abellán, et al., "Timing of food intake predicts weight loss effectiveness," *International Journal of Obesity* (2013): 37, 604–611/doi.10.1038/ijo.2012.229.

CHAPTER 8

A. A. Welch, A. J. MacGregor, et al., "A higher alkaline dietary load is associated with greater indexes of skeletal muscle mass in women," *Osteoporosis International* (2013): 24 (6):1899-908.doi:1007/s00198 -012-2203-7.

R. E. Taylor-Pilliae, W. L. Haskell, et al., "Improvement in balance, strength, and flexibility after 12 weeks of tai chi exercise in ethnic Chinese adults with cardiovascular disease risk factors," *Alternative Therapies in Health and Medicine* (2006): 12 (2): 50–58.

CHAPTER 9

A. E.-Son Om and Kyung-Won Chung, "Dietary Zinc Deficiency Alters 5a-Reduction and Aromatization of Testosterone and Androgen and Estrogen Receptors in Rat Liver," *Journal of Nutrition* (1996), http://in.nutrition.org/content.126/4/842.full pdf+html.

Katharina Buck, Alda Karina Zainedden, et al., "Meta-analyses of lignans and enterolignans in relation to breast cancer risk," *American Journal of Clinical Nutrition* (July 2010): ajcn.28573.

CHAPTER 10

Rebecca Seguin, PhD, CSCS; David M. Buchner, MD, MPH; et al., "Sedentary Behavior and Mortality in Older Women," *American Journal of Preventive Medicine* vol. 46, no. 2 (February 2014): 122– 135.

Maike Neuhaus, MPsych; Genevieve N. Healy, PhD; et al., "Workplace Sitting and Height-Adjustable Workstations, *American Journal of Preventive Medicine* vol. 46, no. 1 (January 2014): 30–40.

Alpa V. Patel, Leslie Bernstein, et al., "Leisure Time Spent Sitting in Relation to Total Mortality in a Prospective Cohort of US Adults, *American Journal of Epidemiology* (2010): 172 (4): 419–429. doi:10.1093 /aje/kwq155.

CHAPTER 11

Riley Bove, MD; Elizabeth Secor; et al., "Early Surgical Menopause Associated with a Spectrum of Cognitive Decline," Findings reported at 2013 meeting of the American Academy of Neurology (2013).

CHAPTER 12

Global Change, University of Michigan, "History of Genetically Modified Foods," www.globalchange.umich.edu/globalchange2/current/workspace/sect008/s8g5/history.htm.

"GMO Fight Ripples Down the Food Chain" by Annie Gasparro, *Wall Street Journal* (August 7, 2014): 1.

Erin S. LeBlanc, MD, MPH; Nancy Perrin, PhD; et al., "Over-the-Counter and Compounded Vitamin D: Is Potency What We Expect? *JAMA Internal Medicine* (2013): 173 (7): 585–586, doi:10.1001/jamainternmed.2013.3812.

"Multivitamins Put to the Test; Defects Found in Nearly 40% Chosen for Review," Product Review (April 9, 2013), www.consumerlab.com.

Steven G. Newmaster, Meghan Grguric, et al., "DNA barcoding detects contamination and substitution in North American herbal products," *BMC Medicine* (2013): 11:222, doi:10.1186/1741-7015-11-222.

Resources

American Academy of Anti-Aging Medicine, http://www.a4m.com

American Association of Naturopathic Physicians (AANP), http://www
.americannaturopathic.org

American Naturopaths Association, http://www.americannaturopaths
association.com

Anti-Anxiety Food Solution, http://www.antianxietyfoodsolution.com

Dr. Robyn Benson, www.robynbenson.com

Cabeca Health, www.cabecahealth.com

Environmental Working Group, http://www.ewg.org

Luminosity, http://www.luminosity.com

Amy Medling, www.pcosdiva.com

My Menopause Magazine, www.mymenopausemagazine.com

National Osteoporosis Association, http://nof.org

Non GMO Project, http://www.nongmoproject.org

PCOS Foundation, http://www.PCOSfoundation.org

Dr. Kellyann Petrucci, http://drkellyann.com/

SpectraCell Laboratories, http://www.spectracell.com

Summer BOCK, www.summerbock.com

U.S. Pharmacopoeial Convention, http://www.usp.org/usp-verification
-services/usp-verified-dietary-supplements/consumers

Village Green Apothecary, www.myvillagegreen.com

Regularly check my website drtami.com for my weekly blog with the latest information on hormones and health. For help with planning nutrient-dense meals, see http://fk152.isrefer.com/go/savingdinner /drtami/.

Index

hormone replacement, *see* bioidentical
hormones; synthetic hormones
hormones, 3–4, 13–32
    aging and, 220
    balance of, 4, 13–14, 230
    decline in levels of, 2–3, 4
    liver and, 101–4, 148
    self-test for level of, 6
    sex, 4, 103
    steroid, 75, 103
    see also specific hormones
hormones, boosting and balancing, 14,
        51–71, 145–46, 173–90, 215
    increasing hormone activity without
        increasing hormone amount,
        51–52
    see also estrogen, boosting and
        balancing; progesterone,
        boosting and balancing;
        testosterone, boosting and
        balancing
hot flashes, 15, 16, 60, 63–64, 67, 68, 219
hummus, 130
    Papa's traditional, 140–41
hypothyroidism, 98
    self-test for, 99
hysterectomy, 44–45, 48, 182, 220
    estrogen and, 19–20
    hormone replacement for, 229–31
    testosterone and, 27–28

I
IgA cells, 135
infertility, 179, 189
inflammation, 3, 29, 39, 77, 78, 80–81,
        88, 89, 119
    cholesterol and, 70, 114
    food allergies and, 135
insulin, 29–30, 53, 123
insulin resistance, 30, 34
iodine, 94, 98–100, 166
iron, 124, 253
isoflavonoids, 64

J
juicing, 108, 127, 150, 152–54, 195–97, 213

K
kefir, 132–33

L
lasagna, Rocco's, 199–201
laughter, 96
lavender, 94, 208
lecithin, 109
legumes, 64, 182
lemon juice, 125
levothyroxine, 231
libido, *see* sex life
licorice root, 95, 166
lignans, 64, 182–83
liver, 7, 24, 101, 119
    alcohol and, 106, 110–11
    cancer and, 101
    chemicals and, 102, 115, 148
    cholesterol and, 113–15
    emotions and, 102, 110–12
    fatty, 115–16
    hormones and, 101–4, 148
    medications and, 111
    signs of problems with, 103
    thyroid and, 115
liver cleanse, 7, 101–17, 125, 145,
        147–57, 185
    body treatments in, 105, 154–55
    daily food schedule for, 149–50
    difficulty of, 113
    exercise and, 156
    foods in, 106, 150–51
    herbs in, 108–9
    juicing in, 127, 150, 152–54
    nutrition guidelines for, 148–54
    substances and conditions to watch
        out for during, 107
    supplements for, 155
    taking care of yourself during, 156
    timing of, 112–13, 156–57

liver-function test (LFT), 103, 248–49
lunch, 115, 128–29, 149, 162, 164, 193

M

maca, 7, 57, 176, 181, 207
magnesium, 94, 155, 166
malnourishment, 120, 124
manganese, 94, 166
marshmallow root, 108
meals, 121
 breakfast, 115, 123, 125–28, 149,
  163–64, 192, 205
 dinner, 115, 130–31, 150, 162,
  165, 193, 203
 eating with intention, 136, 203
 lunch, 115, 128–29, 149, 162, 164,
  193
 in restaurants and while traveling,
  204–5
 snacks, 88, 121, 128, 129–30, 131,
  149, 160, 164, 165, 192, 193, 205
meat, 131
 hormones in, 3, 69
 organic, 69
 protein in, 56
medications:
 estrogen and, 68
 grapefruit and, 107, 111, 151–52
 liver and, 111
 supplements and, 57, 66
 testosterone and, 68
MediClear, 155
meditation, 82–85, 170, 208, 209–14
 Holosync, 84–85, 170, 208, 212
 tai chi, 86, 171–72, 209, 212
 Transcendental Meditation, 83,
  209–12
melatonin, 61–62, 85, 208–9
memory, 4, 41, 230
 Alzheimer's disease and, 5, 42–43
 brain fog and, 23
 estrogen and, 18–20
 phosphatidylcholine and, 109

menopause, 2, 4, 13–18, 50, 255
 surgical, *see* hysterectomy
menorrhagia, 67
menstruation, 18
 progesterone and, 24
micronutrients, 52–53, 124, 194, 252–53
milk thistle, 108–9, 155
mindfulness, 83
minerals, 7, 119
 adrenals and, 93–94, 166
 boron, 67, 181
 calcium, 47, 93, 166
 chromium, 94, 166
 copper, 59, 94, 166, 253
 estrogen and, 67, 180
 iodine, 94, 98–100, 166
 iron, 124, 253
 magnesium, 94, 155, 166
 manganese, 94, 166
 molybdenum, 94, 166
 selenium, 70, 94, 155, 166, 188
 synergies and, 253
 testosterone and, 56–59, 177
 trace, 94, 166
 zinc, 58–59, 67, 155, 166, 176,
  177, 181, 253
miscarriages, 23–24, 187
molybdenum, 94, 166
mood, 4, 41
 irritability, 15, 24, 187
movement, 97–98, 213–15
 see also exercise
mucuna pruriens, 57–58
muesli, 123
 Dr. Tami's morning, 138
muscles, 125, 162, 220
muscle-to-fat ratio, 4, 9, 34–35, 36

N

NASH (nonalcoholic steatohepatitis),
 115–16
naturopaths, 243–44
Nexium, 111

My website is an important resource for my patients and readers, so I invite you to check out drtami.com to become a part of *The Hormone Secret* community and gain access to the latest information on hormones and health. You can take my free Hormone Quiz and receive your personal Hormone Secret Handbook, with individualized recommendations for your health and wellness. Don't forget to sign up for my email newsletter and subscribe to my blog so you can receive the latest health news alongside exclusive features and tips!

As a reader of my book, visit drtami.com/bookbonus to learn how to receive access to your special bonus material:

- An exclusive cookbook by Dr. Tami featuring fifty healthy, delicious recipes that will help naturally balance your hormone levels
- An exclusive workout video guest-starring a surprise fitness celebrity